SURVIVING THE

MENTAL HEALTH TANK

Surviving the Mental Health Tank

Five Keys to Cultivating Emotional Well-Being for Yourself and Your Loved Ones

BY TAMU LEWIS

ISBN: 979-8-9862677-0-8

Table of Contents

Introduction: The Lives We Choose to Lead · · · · · · · · · · · · · vii

Chapter 1   Defining the Tank· 1
Chapter 2   Surviving the Tank · 15
Chapter 3   Letting Go of Control (First Key) · · · · · · · · · · · 33
Chapter 4   Don't Take It Personally (Second Key) · · · · · · · 51
Chapter 5   From Grief to Healing (Third Key)· · · · · · · · · · 61
Chapter 6   Manage Your Expectations (Fourth Key)· · · · · · 75
Chapter 7   Intentional Self-Care (Fifth Key)· · · · · · · · · · · 91
Chapter 8   Education Is Key· 107
Chapter 9   Setting Up a Lifetime Management and
              Treatment Plan · 119

Conclusion· 135
Glossary of Terms · 141
About the Author· 149

INTRODUCTION
The Lives We Choose to Lead

There are only four kinds of people in the world:
those who have been caregivers, those who are
currently caregivers, those who will be caregivers,
and those who will need a caregiver.
—Rosalyn Carter

JOHN LENNON ONCE SAID, "Life is what happens to you while you're busy making other plans." He certainly could have been talking about me. I was gliding along, running my consulting business, and taking care of my family when my life took an abrupt turn.

At that point, I knew very little about bipolar disorder. I had no idea how it would impact my life. If you are as innocent and uninformed as I was, let me offer some surprising facts.

Although the average American often doesn't know the term, bipolar disorder affects millions of Americans. Unless we are close to someone who has been diagnosed with bipolar disorder, we have little or no idea what it's really like to live with it or to live with someone who is affected by it.

For once in the history of medical terminology, the term *bipolar* accurately describes the condition. There are extreme highs interspersed with extreme lows. One day someone with bipolar disorder might be manic, and the next day they might be extremely depressed. Moods can change from minute to minute. While these symptoms usually alternate, they may also occur at the same time.

Here's an example: If you suffer from bipolar disorder, you may feel full of energy and optimism, yet you might also feel anxious and be unable to sit still. A week later, you could feel ill, exhausted, lethargic, and apathetic. This would be a low or depressive episode. Mixed episodes of mania and depression are doubly confusing for the entire family. The outward appearance or symptoms of bipolar disorder can vary greatly from one person to the next. Some people are able to mask their symptoms so that those on the outside looking in would never guess the person has bipolar disorder. For others, the challenges of living with and managing bipolar disorder are more evident.

Some of us worry about bipolar disorder when other family members suffer from it. While you don't catch bipolar disorder like you do a cold or the flu, it does have a tendency to run in families. This has strengthened the myth that it's contagious.

Another myth is that people are born with bipolar disorder. It's typically not diagnosed in young children and usually appears during late teen years or early twenties. Bipolar disorder is especially hard to diagnose in children and teenagers. Some of this difficulty lies in the fact that, as their brains are developing, kids naturally experience highs and lows. But their moods just aren't as extreme as those of kids diagnosed as bipolar. The line between normal and bipolar is often blurry in children and adolescents. With kids, symptoms tend to be severe, violent fits followed by happy, over-the-top times. In teens, it may show up as reckless behavior, a sudden drop in grades and disinterest in activities they previously loved.

Another complication in identifying bipolar disorder in this age group is the fact that the signs and symptoms can and often do overlap with symptoms of other disorders common in young people. These include attention-deficit hyperactivity disorder (ADHD), conduct problems, major depression, and anxiety disorders.

Diagnosing bipolar disorder is complicated. It requires a careful and thorough evaluation by a trained, experienced mental health expert. Labeling a child's problem as bipolar disorder is both a gift and a curse, so it is important to get it right. Once diagnosed, children may have an Individualized Education Program (IEP) outlining the special needs they require medically and academically in order to prosper. If the diagnosis is wrong, the interventions may be ineffective or even harmful.

There is no cure for bipolar disorder. It's a condition you and your loved ones have to manage and live with. Bipolar disorder requires a lifetime management and treatment plan. In a later chapter, we will discuss what experts have to say about setting up a lifetime management and treatment plan. We'll also share how several families have turned this into reality.

My aim in sharing my experiences in dealing with bipolar disorder and other mental health challenges in my family is to help others who share this struggle. My wish is that my story will bring you hope and reassurance.

Later we'll address misinformation around bipolar disorder and the harm arising from these myths.

CHAPTER 1
Defining the Tank

Emotional pain is not something that should be
hidden away and never spoken about. There is
truth in your pain, there is growth in your pain, but
only if it's first brought out into the open.
—Steven Aitchison

THIS IS THE BEGINNING of the mental health tank. The
tank is symbolic because I felt overwhelmed dealing with all of
the mental health challenges that life was throwing at me. It felt
as if I were drowning in a mental health tank. I'll explain more
about that later. For now, I'll give you a little background as to
what happened and how I made it to this point.

I was the first child born to two parents. Everyone looked
forward to my arrival, and I was welcomed with love. I was the
first grandchild on my mom's side. I have fond memories of my
childhood. I would spend a couple weeks every summer with each
set of my grandparents. On my dad's side, I visited Pittsburgh,
Pennsylvania. On my mom's side, I spent time in York, South

Carolina. Everything was great from my perspective...until it wasn't.

When I was seven, my parents divorced. I was heartbroken. I felt very alone. I had always asked for a sibling and did not have one at that point.

Fast forward some years: both of my parents were in new relationships, and my mom gave me a little brother, Lee. He was born when I was twelve. At that point, I was accustomed to being an only child. Having a sibling was an adjustment. Nevertheless, I loved him dearly. I became the live-in babysitter, big sister, chauffeur, and junior mom. It was great.

Lee was a wonderful, bright, intelligent, and curious little guy who looked up to me, his big sister. I would take him with me on various outings because I had to. My mom's expectation was that I would be responsible and help take care of Lee. He was with me at high school basketball games. I drove him to tae kwon do and picked him up from school when needed. I remember asking my mom if she could make Lee stop talking. He was an entertainer at heart, so he was always talking, telling stories, and entertaining anyone who would listen.

When I left to go to college, Lee was five and I was seventeen. He was very sad. We asked him why he was so sad, and he said it was because his big sister and all of his friends were leaving for college. My friends were his friends, and he was only five. In hindsight, I realized that my going off to college was a stressful, traumatic event for him.

At that point, I was starting my journey to becoming a college student and young adult. I was learning how to take care of myself. I graduated from the University of South Carolina with a BS in finance and went to work at a major financial institution. I had a good, professional job. Then I chose to go to graduate school at the University of North Carolina to get an MBA.

That all went well. I graduated and met someone with whom I became very good friends. Eventually, friendship turned to love. That good friend became my husband; we were married in 2000. We adopted a child in 2002 and then had a child in 2004. I would say that my life was going along pretty much as expected...until it wasn't.

I received a call from my mom during the summer of 2003, explaining that my brother had had some type of episode involving mental health challenges. This was the summer between Lee's senior year in high school and his first year of college. He was eighteen at the time. She took him to a psychiatrist. There was no official diagnosis. I just remember them saying he needed a lot of rest to reset.

It didn't seem like that big of a deal. It may have been the way she explained it or my perception of the situation. Admittedly, I was distracted by the events of my personal life. At the time, I lacked any sort of mental health education. Perhaps that made Lee's situation seem minor. Years later I would learn that Lee had been traveling, and upon his return to New York, he couldn't find his luggage or wallet and couldn't find his way home.

I think the episode occurred over a few days. Then, within a week or so, from what I could tell, it seemed like everything was back to normal. At this point, Lee and my mom were living in New York; I was living in Atlanta.

Lee went on to attend the University of Southern California and graduated magna cum laude with a BA in cinema and television. He was also in a couple of major movies (*Akeelah and the Bee* and *Friday Night Lights*). If I recall correctly, my brother had another episode. But again, it didn't seem like a big deal. I remember thinking he was probably stressed out and putting too much pressure on himself.

In 2007, Lee was twenty-three. He called and didn't sound like himself. He knew he was dealing with some type of imbalance. He was paranoid. He was in LA, and my mom and I were on the East Coast. My mom flew out to LA. I talked with him on the phone for several hours to keep him grounded until she arrived. I was traveling in Greenville, South Carolina with my husband and two daughters at the time. Lee said that my voice was calming. I ordered food for him because he was too paranoid to go outside. I had him watch a comedy movie. My mom got a referral for a psychiatrist in LA. My mom stayed in LA with Lee for a couple of weeks until he was stable enough to fly. The LA psychiatrist gave Lee the diagnosis of bipolar disorder. Lee flew back to Florida with my mom and stayed for a few weeks to aid in his recovery.

The term *bipolar* meant little to me. So, like all smart people, I googled it. Here is what I discovered:

- One of the defining characteristics of bipolar disorder is, as the name suggests, dramatic shifts in mood and behavior. These are called mood episodes.

- Bipolar lows look a lot like clinical depression and are often misdiagnosed and treated as depression.

- Bipolar highs or manic episodes might show up as pronounced activity, unusually high energy, looking and acting jumpy, irritability, overconfidence, insomnia, rapid speech, or risky behavior.

- Manic episodes may last up to a week or more. Serious episodes may require hospitalization.

- It is not uncommon to have mixed episodes of highs and lows.

- Bipolar disorder is not just one thing. There are four types: Bipolar I is characterized by sharp mood swings and up to two weeks of manic and depressive episodes. Bipolar II sufferers experience depression and hypomania—not full mania. Bipolar III is cyclothymia—a less severe form of the disorder. Left untreated, cyclothymia can develop into I or II. Finally, Bipolar IV symptoms are so mild that they are deemed unspecified bipolar disorder.

- Bipolar disorder may make it difficult or impossible to carry out daily living tasks.

Armed with this information, I traveled to Florida from Georgia with my daughters and stayed for a week to help support my mom and brother. I wanted to help in any way possible to ensure that my brother would be okay.

This is where I first began to have some level of understanding of mental illness, particularly bipolar disorder. As I mentioned earlier, my brother was brilliant. He was a successful, working actor with roles in different movies and TV shows. I believe his brilliance helped him mask the illness a lot of the time. He spent a lot of time being well, or at least appearing well.

I think that played a part in my ignorance around the seriousness of mental health challenges. At that time, my brother's mental health challenges didn't appear to be ongoing. He was under the care of a psychiatrist. He did talk therapy as well, and things seem to be managed.

For those unfamiliar with talk therapy, it involves discussing your thoughts, feelings, concerns, and behaviors with a trained professional. By describing what's going on in your head and how that makes you feel, you can identify behaviors you may want to change.

Also known as psychotherapy, talk therapy is effective in treatment of bipolar disorder. It helps build an understanding and, hopefully, a mastery of behaviors that interfere with social and work situations.

In Lee's case, there appeared to be years between his episodes. As Lee matured into an adult, he seemed aware of when an imbalance was taking place. When they occurred, he would call me or my mom.

Sometimes, we would talk to him together on a three-way call. We would figure out what needed to be done. I would go to LA, my mom would make the trip, or a close relative would go. We would talk to his psychiatrist and stay in LA until he stabilized.

Lee's episodes were never severe enough to require hospitalization. It seemed like we could always identify a trigger when an imbalance and episode would occur.

It is important to understand and identify bipolar disorder triggers. By understanding certain triggers, you can better manage bipolar disorder for yourself or a family member.

One of the most common triggers is stress. This can be caused by a traumatic event or situation, such as an exam. While changes in sleep patterns are a symptom of bipolar disorder, they can also be a trigger. Breakups and arguments may trigger bipolar episodes.

While alcohol or drug use don't cause bipolar disorder, they can certainly trigger episodes. Taking antidepressants can control a low episode, but they may trigger a manic episode.

Each time, once my brother was stabilized, we would return to our own respective homes and lives, thinking all was well... until it wasn't.

The last time that an episode occurred was in February 2013. At that point, Lee was filming a TV show. He had never missed a day of work. He called and said that he needed one of us to come to LA. My mom had just lost a dear friend and needed to attend the funeral. So I went to LA to help Lee. Fortunately, I have a husband who is able and willing to hold down the home front with our two daughters whenever I have to travel.

I traveled to LA and stayed with Lee for about a week. While I was there, he never missed a day of work. I went to Paramount Studios with him each day, and he nailed his lines like the consummate, professional actor he was. From the outside looking in, I thought he seemed fine. I was in contact with his psychiatrist, and we worked through things regarding Lee's medication and routine.

Those dealing with bipolar disorder most often have medicines to control the highs and lows. These are called mood stabilizers. One of the most prescribed drugs for bipolar disorder is lithium. It is the cornerstone of treatment both for mania and depression. Lithium is the oldest and best-known mood stabilizer and is highly effective for treating mania. Because bipolar disorder is a lifelong condition, treatment may change as symptoms change. Treatment is aimed at managing symptoms. Besides medication, treatment may include day treatment programs that offer support and counseling to get symptoms under control. Groups that focus on education or support are often helpful.

Finding the right medication or medications takes some trial and error. This process requires patience, as it may take weeks or months for the medication to take full effect. Doctors usually change only one medication at a time in order to identify which medications work to relieve unique symptoms or side effects. As symptoms change, medications may need to be readjusted. The entire procedure is a balancing act. It can be very frustrating.

Unfortunately, those with bipolar disorder sometimes make changes or stop taking their medications without a doctor's recommendation. They think they no longer need it, or they don't like the side effects. Changes in medication can cause withdrawal effects, or bipolar symptoms may worsen or return.

To help us both feel grounded and stable during those challenging times, I also did meditation with Lee. Then, as usual, I returned home when he seemed to be feeling better.

In July 2013, I happened to be traveling to Hawaii with my husband and some friends for a vacation. Lee was on vacation in Hawaii at the same time, even though we had not planned it. We were able to connect, have dinner, and spend some time together in Hawaii. Little did I know, that would be the last time I saw Lee.

On August 19, 2013, I received a call that Lee had not shown up on set to film the TV show. That was very unlike him. As I mentioned earlier, he had never missed a day of work. The call was from his manager, asking if I had spoken with him that weekend, and I had not. The last conversation I'd had with him was about a week before. We both tried calling, and there was no answer. Lee's manager went to his building and had security access Lee's apartment.

They found him. He had died by suicide. This was obviously the last episode, and Lee was able to mask it until the suicide. We had not heard any signs in his voice.

The reason that I share this experience is because Lee kept his diagnosis to himself. As far as I know, only a few people were aware of his bipolar disorder diagnosis. His friends, coworkers, and other family members did not know. He was living alone in LA while my mom and I were living in our respective homes on the East Coast. I feel that if there wasn't such a stigma around mental illness and Lee had been able to share his diagnosis, his community may have noticed signs.

It is sadly usual for those with bipolar disorder to feel stigmatized. People diagnosed with bipolar disorder are often discriminated against when others know their diagnosis. They often feel stigmatized at work. Attitudes of family members and their prejudices toward those with mental illnesses often keep those with bipolar disorder silent about their condition. We're going to talk seriously about the stigma surrounding bipolar disorder and the harm it can cause in a later chapter.

Understanding bipolar disorder is further complicated by the fact that no two individuals share the same symptoms, behaviors, or social experiences. Medications and side effects often vary widely. It should, therefore, come as no surprise that coping with bipolar disorder also varies. Lee tended to carry on as if everything was fine. His cries for help to me and my mom were limited. His coworkers had no idea about the toll his manic and depressive phases were taking on him.

Sadly, too many of those who suffer from bipolar disorder see it not as an illness but as a sign of personal weakness. This jeopardizes their ability to cope. Bipolar disorder is a health condition just like diabetes, kidney failure, or heart disease. We need to get this message out to those who are diagnosed with bipolar disorder (or other mental illnesses) and to those around them. I will share initiatives other loved ones have put forth to address this problem of self-blame or survivor's guilt.

Bipolar disorder stigma, as with that of many other mental illnesses, comes mainly from a lack of understanding of the condition. We humans fear what we don't understand. For me, learning about bipolar helped not only Lee but also others around him. I vowed after Lee's tragic end that I would do everything in my power to educate my family, friends, and community about mental illness. Building awareness will be empowering for us all. In a later chapter, I will talk about how rewarding it is to raise awareness about mental illness. You, too, can become a mental health advocate.

In hindsight, when I spoke with some of his coworkers, they told me that Lee didn't seem like himself at rehearsal, but he performed fine. When they asked him how he was doing, he just said he was tired, and they accepted his answer. However, if you have awareness about mental illness and you know someone has a diagnosis or they have mental health challenges, if they say they're tired, you may respond differently. You may ask how you can be supportive and helpful. Being supportive may just involve being there and listening or reaching out for help on that person's behalf if needed.

It is important for me to share my experiences, increase mental health awareness, and work to erase the stigma associated with mental illness. Mental illness takes place in the brain, which is an organ in our bodies just like the other organs of the human body. However, mental illness is oftentimes invisible unless there is an active episode occurring.

POEM: WHAT I NOW KNOW

What I now know is…
when we were listening to "The Good Life" in your living room,
your life wasn't "good" and hadn't been for a while.

What I now know is…
when you were acting on TV and saying your lines just right,
you were also acting in real life, trying to hold on tight.

Trying to hold on to your family,
trying to hold on to your friends,
trying to hold on to your faith, your heart, and your art.

You fought a good fight, my dear.
It allowed us to hold you near…at least for a while.

And during the time that you were here,
you did more for others than most do over a lifetime of years.

You left your mark, my dear brother.
Your light lives on through others.

Together, we will make a difference
in hopes that so many others won't suffer.

…At least not in silence.

Then we can all learn more from one another.
So we can do more for each other.

And our lights can shine on…

Useful Resources

Aimee Daramus, *Understanding Bipolar Disorder: The Essential Family Guide,* (Emeryville: Rockridge Press, 2020)

Kostas Fountoulakis, *Bipolar Disorder: An Evidence-Based Guide to Dealing with Manic Depression,* (Thessaloniki: Springer, 2014)

David J. Miklowitz, PhD and Michael J. Gitlin, MD, *Clinician's Guide to Bipolar Disorder,* (New York: The Guilford Press, 2015)

Vivek H. Murthy, *Together: The Healing Power of Human Connection in a Sometimes Lonely World,* (New York: Harper Wave, 2020)

Michael Rose, *Bipolar Wellness,* (Gainesville: Bipolar Wellness Press, 2018)

Ruth C. White and John D. Preston, *Bipolar 101,* (Oakland: New Harbinger Publications, 2008)

CHAPTER 2
Surviving the Tank

WHEN WE LEFT OFF in Chapter 1, I was explaining how I got into the tank. My oldest daughter, Nya, began to act out at school. She was at a public charter school at the time, and she had a 504 Plan for accommodations that would help her manage.

For those of you who are unfamiliar with a 504 Plan, it is developed to ensure that a child who is attending an elementary or secondary school and is identified under the law as having a disability receives accommodations aimed at ensuring their academic success and has full access to an effective learning environment. Depending on where you are from, you may be more familiar with the term IEP, which stands for Individualized Education Program. For students with disabilities who require specialized instruction, an IEP is developed under the Individuals with Disabilities Education Act. Both a 504 Plan and an IEP offer plans for accommodations to meet a student's special needs. Basically, the difference is that an IEP provides students from kindergarten to twelfth grade with specialized instruction, while a 504 Plan covers students from kindergarten through college.

Here are some examples of 504 Plan accommodations:

- Seating in a particular space in the classroom

- Extended time to take tests or complete assignments

- Reduction in homework or classroom assignments

- Use of technological aids

- Behavior modification programs

- Modified texts or specialized audio-video materials

- Behavior management techniques

- Oral testing

- Permission to move to quiet area or room when the classroom gets too noisy or crowded

Nya was in the sixth grade. The teachers were losing patience with her behavior. She was being put outside of the classroom a lot. At that point in Nya's life, the school no longer served our needs. We realized that the passing of my brother had been very difficult for her, and we had to step up in terms of the frequency of visits to Nya's psychiatrist for talk therapy. We had weekly appointments for intensive therapy for about eight weeks to try to break her out of the rut that she was in. The psychiatrist was very helpful, giving Nya writing exercises to help her process her feelings about losing her Uncle Lee. My younger daughter, Kai, was in shock and at that time didn't really believe that Lee had died. Thus, Nya felt like she couldn't talk to Kai about her feelings. I also think Nya was trying to protect me and didn't want to share her feelings with me because she knew that I was having a hard time with the loss of my brother.

I began a search of various types of public, private, and hybrid schools to find a better fit for Nya. Eventually, we found a private school that was equipped to deal with Nya's special needs. It had little diversity, but it provided a lot of the support that Nya needed. While I was waiting for Nya to finish a group therapy session for teens, I was reading a newsletter from the school that she would eventually attend. I remember thinking: *This seems like a great place.*

The school had an open house day scheduled for prospective families. My husband, Stephen, was already scheduled to be out of town on a business trip that day. I called Nya's godmother, Lasaundra, and asked her to come with me. She said, "Count me in. I'll be there."

It was great to have the support of my close friend. I knew that I needed someone to be with me. I didn't want to assess the school by myself. I was so impressed and moved by the open house activities. I felt like crying tears of relief and joy. In fact, I think I did cry once I was alone. Student testimonials and performances were part of the program that day.

I remember tearing up for sure while watching the students perform. I'm a sucker for musical and theatrical performances. Nya started attending the school at the beginning of her seventh-grade year. She attended seventh and eighth grade at MSA. The school's learning environment was a better fit for her. Nya earned excellent grades. She even played on the girls' basketball team during her eighth-grade year.

The social aspect was still a struggle. Often the public does not understand that children who suffer with bipolar disorder get more excited and agitated than others their age. They go through cycles of extreme highs and lows. These mood changes affect their relationships with others at home and school.

Bipolar mood changes are more extreme. They are also often unprovoked. Mood changes are often accompanied by changes in sleep patterns. Energy levels and the ability to think clearly are often affected. Bipolar symptoms often make it difficult for kids Nya's age to do well in school. It is also hard for them to get along with friends and family. Our greatest fear was that, like Lee, Nya would hurt herself or attempt suicide.

This isn't just panic or paranoia talking when I mention suicide. Studies have shown that the attempted suicide rate of youth with bipolar disorder is between 20 and 45 percent. The greatest suicide age risk is youth in general, and bipolar disorder raises that risk. Of those who attempt, between 10 and 20 percent will complete the act. Factors studied include a history of suicide attempts, a family history of suicide, mood swings, depressive polarity, rapidly fluctuating mood changes, frequent hospitalization, or frequent unsuccessful medication changes.

I began receiving weekly calls from the school about some type of behavioral issue Nya was having. The school was located about thirty minutes from our house. Sometimes the trip took longer depending on traffic. I found myself having to go to Nya's school more often than I would have liked to discuss her behavioral issues. We were paying the tuition out of pocket, and it was very expensive. If this wasn't a successful learning experience for Nya, then perhaps it was time for a change.

At the end of Nya's eighth-grade year, I decided to try the public high school located down the street from our house. My reasoning was that if I was going to get frequent calls about behavioral issues from her expensive private school, I might as well try the free public school close to my house. So that was what we did. The money savings were significant, but it brought more issues. The social aspect was much more challenging in the public school setting due to a higher population of students and higher student-teacher ratios. There was a lot more to navigate compared to the "special needs" school.

Nya began to seek validation from friends who didn't necessarily have her best interests at heart. At some point during her freshman year, she was suspended for fighting with another girl. Nevertheless, Nya made it through her freshman year.

As her sophomore year began, Nya continued to act out in various ways at school. There were times when she skipped class and times when she threatened to take her own life. Given our experience with Lee and the high rate of teen suicides, we took these threats very seriously. Our challenging times included calling 911 when Nya was a danger to herself. This led to a hospital stay followed by intensive outpatient therapy.

Eventually, we decided that public school was not the best environment for Nya. Fortunately, we were able to return to the private school setting two months into Nya's sophomore year of high school.

We tried multiple approaches and therapies with Nya through the years. These included alternative and traditional therapies and even spiritual techniques. When she was younger, we tried play therapy, natural supplements, breathing techniques, reinforcing good behavior, and implementing consequences for bad behavior. As Nya got older, she received cognitive behavior therapy (CBT) and dialectical behavior therapy (DBT), both individual and group, throughout high school.

CBT is a treatment intervention aimed at improving mental health. It focuses on changing behaviors by teaching coping strategies. In most cases, CBT is a gradual process that helps a person take incremental steps toward a behavior change. The process involves several steps. Here is an example: If someone has society anxiety, the first step might be visualizing situations that would cause anxiety for that person. The next step might be practicing dialogue with their therapist. This could be followed by practicing conversations with friends, coworkers, or family members.

CBT is rooted in how we think, feel, and consequently behave. The belief is that thoughts determine our feelings and thus our behavior. Anxiety is caused by negative and unrealistic thoughts that can cause us distress and result in problems.

DBT is an evolving medical treatment in which the person accepts the reality of a situation and decides how they will change it. DBT emphasizes interpersonal relations. Techniques include the following:

- Mindfulness—becoming aware of and accepting the present situation

- Distress tolerance—handling those crises that mindfulness can't cope with

- Interpersonal effectiveness—dealing with social situations

- Emotion regulation—keeping reactions in check

Both CBT and DBT include talk therapy. The aim is to better understand and manage one's thoughts and reactions. DBT emphasizes managing emotions and dealing with relationships. It is effective in working with those who have bipolar disorder because dramatic mood swings make relationships challenging.

Even with all of the treatments and therapeutic techniques we tried, we still experienced some episodes and hospitalizations, along with a lot of disruption in our household. There were times when I felt like one of us wasn't going to make it through those challenging situations. I was in therapy just to maintain my sanity, to be able to parent Nya and my other daughter, and to take care of myself.

Initially, I was resentful. I felt like she had the problem, not me. But I soon discovered that her problems were my problems.

This was causing issues for me as an adult. I felt betrayed. "We adopted her at five months old," I was saying. "Why would God give us this child if she wasn't going to accept our help?"

It was exhausting and heartbreaking. Eventually, I realized the dreams I had for her were my dreams, not hers. Her dreams were different. I learned to support her.

During her senior year, we hit a really rough patch. Nya fell into a deep depression. It was so severe that she was not able to get out of bed most days. Nya was contemplating dropping out of high school.

The approaches that we had learned in terms of setting boundaries and helping her to feel motivated were not working. We were fortunate enough to find an in-home family therapy program. We were initially on the waitlist for about two weeks. If space in the program wasn't available, I considered liquidating my retirement savings to pay for a therapeutic boarding school if it would help my daughter. I was exploring all options because I felt helpless and very stressed out about the situation.

We began the in-home therapy program for our whole family, not just for Nya. The therapist would first meet briefly with Stephen and me for an update on anything that happened since our previous session. Then the therapist would meet with Nya alone. At the end of each in-home session, we would all meet with the therapist to work through any challenges and discuss next steps. Nya was very resistant at first. However, the counselor, Christina, was consistent and calm. She showed up every week. Initially, those sessions may have been twice a week.

Once Nya realized that Christina wasn't going anywhere and was going to keep showing up, Nya slowly began to open up to her. Christina was able to pull things out of Nya that my husband and I couldn't as her parents. These things helped her feel supported.

I learned that, even though there were things I would say that I thought showed support and love, that was not the way Nya was receiving those messages. Her processing of my words and actions was different from what I thought. With support from Christina, Nya was able to make suggestions about things that we could do as parents. Something as simple as saying, "How are you?" instead of saying, "How was your day?" or "How was school?" could make a big difference for her. In her thought process, Nya was thinking that we cared only about her school and her grades and that we didn't care about her as a person.

Nya was in sixth grade when my brother passed. I didn't realize the deep impact it had on her at the time. I was crushed when I got the call. I had just gone to LA to visit my brother in February 2013 when he had reached out for help.

I left my family during that time to go and stay with him. I did the best I could with the knowledge that I had at the time. I was in contact with his psychiatrist and his spiritual leader. At that time, I felt like I was able to help my brother feel grounded and support him while I was there. He was taking his medications as prescribed. He never missed a day of filming the TV show *Rizzoli and Isles*. So once he was better, I returned home. I happened to see him again in July while we were both vacationing in Hawaii at the same time, unplanned.

On August 19, I received the call. Lee had passed by suicide. It was unthinkable. It was the most horrible thing that I had ever encountered. I blamed myself initially. I thought I had missed something. I thought I should have known. I thought I should have done more. I realized, in hindsight, that Lee was in a lot of pain and suffering in silence. His death made me feel like a piece of my heart had been cut out. He was my little brother, born when I was twelve. I was his protector. Now I had to bury him and keep myself together to raise my two daughters.

Everything was painful. Sometimes I couldn't breathe. Sometimes I was deeply depressed. I had to go to a therapist and a psychiatrist to work through the grief myself. When I initially scheduled the appointment the psychiatrist, I knew that my husband would be traveling, and I thought I would be fine going to the appointment alone. I was wrong. Once I got in the car, I realized the gravity of the situation, and I called my cousin Bryan. Fortunately, he was able to meet me at the psychiatrist's office. I remember crying as I was driving to the psychiatrist's office because I didn't want to be in such pain, and I didn't want to "need" medication. I called a friend of mine, Pam, who had lost her mother to suicide. She is an executive and would typically be in meetings during the day; however, she happened to be available when I called. She encouraged me and talked to me all the way to the psychiatrist's office. If she hadn't answered the phone, I'm not sure if I would have made it to the office that day. I ended up having to take medication for depression for a period of time just to keep it all together and be able to function on a daily basis. It was a struggle. I felt like I was being punished, and I was the one who had stayed. I felt sick. I felt like I was going to die from an illness. I was broken.

With help from my therapist, psychiatrist, friends, and family, I made it through. I pulled myself together.

My tribe came out to take me to dinner on my side of town. I couldn't articulate how bad I was feeling. One of my girlfriends came over when I didn't feel like getting out of bed. She just came over and sat in the bed with me. I don't know what my husband was feeling at the time, but he was probably thinking, *Whatever helps, you do it.*

My childhood best friend came to visit from Alabama to just sit and talk and take me to the movies for a distraction. My family took me to the beach to do a cleanse. They did prayer circles. We had a certain day of the week where we would have a call early in the morning. People would pray for me on that call. I prayed and cried a lot and journaled to voice my feelings. I even wrote poetry. I don't consider myself to be a poet. Almost immediately after my brother's death, my mom and I cofounded a nonprofit organization, the Lee Thompson Young Foundation. The organization's mission is to promote mental health education in schools, communities, and organizations and to help erase the stigma associated with mental illness. I thought my mom and I were going to run it together. However, it ended up being on my shoulders. It was too much to focus on, but I did it because I knew the organization was helping others.

I felt burned out after five years of running the organization while working in my consulting business. I thought about closing the foundation, but the universe sent a wonderful mental health professional to run it. Now I serve as the board president.

Nya's senior year was extremely challenging. COVID-19 hit, and the world was thrust into a pandemic. I knew there had to be a change. We needed space. Of course, a traditional college experience involves moving out and going away to college.

That wasn't a fit for Nya. There was a time when she seriously considered dropping out of high school. The fact that she'd made it through high school and finished with straight A's was a huge accomplishment. She decided to go to a local community college and selected a major that she loves. My husband and I decided we would move her into an apartment nearby so we could support her and she could learn to support herself. Then we could have space in our home for healing and growth. Miraculously, she rose to the occasion. I knew she had it in her to do it, but I didn't believe it until I saw it. I had always hoped that she would thrive as she got older and matured.

Nya went from isolating herself, not wanting to spend time with us, not wanting to eat with us, and not wanting to talk to us to appreciating our family. She comes to visit on her own initiative two to three times a week. And in terms of the things that I would have to battle her to do—like keep a routine, take medication, get enough sleep, be proactive, exercise, and eat right—she is incorporating into her life on her own.

She also knew that once you're eighteen, you don't have to go to counseling. No one can force you to go to any appointments because by law you're an adult. On her own, she decided to continue her talk therapy. Initially, she continued to see her therapist once a week, and now she sees her every other week. She also sees her psychiatrist once a quarter.

She does this on her own. She brings up things that are bothering her that she wants to work on or things she feels may be stressing her out. That's really an accomplishment. I wouldn't believe it if I hadn't seen it myself. Her being able to step up to the plate like that has given me space to step up to the plate as well. I have been able to put a face and a name to the mental health journey and the impact that it can have on a family. Now I can speak out and be a voice for others. I am pleased to act as a resource for others and to help families get through these challenging situations.

Here's something to note: my daughter is very in tune with herself. An alternative medicine practitioner suggested Nya work with animals when she was younger. As a high school freshman, Nya found that working with horses and special needs children made her feel valued, positive, and needed. This led her to choose a major that involved working with animals at the community college. That is grounding for her. She feels needed by the animals. She also has a job working in a doggy day care.

Nya has made decisions that we support. She feels confident and competent. Even when we're not there, knowing that we support her choices gives her a purpose larger than herself. She knows that those animals are counting on her. That helps her show up strong and consistent. I want to emphasize that finding something you love to focus on can be healing by itself. This is a way of focusing on what you love versus what you lack. Like Nya, others have found solace in being around pets.

Those struggling with mental illnesses can often find solace and an easing of their depressed lows and manic highs through their association with service animals or even with "regular" pets. Pet therapy, also known as animal-assisted therapy, is often suggested for those with bipolar disorder or other mood disorders.

Here is how to go about acquiring a service animal: Ask a licensed health care professional to write a letter stating your condition and explaining how an emotional support animal can improve your well-being. The reason this documentation is required has to do with cost and demand. At least two years of intensive training goes into preparing service animals for clients. There is a shortage of service dogs, so only those in great need will qualify.

If you do not qualify or don't want to wait until a service animal is available, consider adopting or purchasing a pet as a companion to help soothe you in challenging times and play with you in happy times.

Here is an example of how beneficial an animal can be: Diane Brody developed high and low mood swings in her twenties. She was going to have to wait over two years for a service animal. So she opted instead to get her own pet. Now Buddy, an Australian border collie, is ten years old.

Buddy has been trained to help Diane deal with problems related to her bipolar disorder. Diane's severe mood swings often result in hallucinations. Buddy helps Diane distinguish between what's real and what's imagined. Buddy is trained to be alert to unusual things around him. This reassures Diane when Buddy doesn't react to her "strange, imagined creatures."

Buddy also helps Diane with her tendency to withdraw. Because Buddy is convinced that everyone is his friend, he makes Diane's walks become social outings.

Service animals can also assist those with mental illnesses in other ways that their owner may require. Below are a few examples:

- Bringing medication or providing reminders to take medication at specific times

- Waking their owner at a specific time each day

- Providing reminders about bedtime; it is vital to keep sleep cycles regular

- Bringing a mobile phone if the owner exhibits alarming behaviors

- Interrupting potentially dangerous behaviors by nudging, nagging, or distracting

- Alerting the owner to the telephone, doorbell, or smoke alarm

- Calming or interrupting manic behaviors

Research shows that pets are a benefit to anyone suffering from mental illness. They offer unconditional love. This does wonders to restore empathy. Here are more examples of what pets can offer:

- Pets help owners feel more connected to the world around them. Their care forces people in social withdrawal to make connections in the neighborhood.

- Pets create a comfortable sense of family in a home.

- Pets build a sense of self-worth and self-confidence. Your life feels more in control when you are responsible for the care and welfare of another.

While pet therapy has many benefits, there are some concerns. Not every dog is cut out to be a therapy dog. Not every animal has the skills or temperament. Not everyone with a mental illness is a pet lover. Owning a therapy pet comes with responsibilities as well as benefits. Not everyone can meet those challenges.

Not every home can accommodate an animal. Some pet therapy risks involve safety and sanitation. Those with allergies to animal dander may have reactions. Keeping the home and animal clean may also be an issue. Some mental illness behaviors may constitute pet abuse.

Therapy and service animals have much they can do for their owners. However, this isn't for everyone. Give careful consideration to the advantages and disadvantages of having a therapy animal before you take this important step.

POEM: ADMIT

I have to admit, at times I felt conflicted.

How could we be celebrating the life that you took from us?

How could we be smiling, remembering the good times, when you are gone?

How could we be cleaning out your place without shedding a tear, deciding what to keep, what to discard, and what to donate?

How could we be planning your memorial services when you were only twenty-nine?

How could we move on when part of our heart was gone?

How could you leave me to handle all of your stuff?

How could we…?

How could you…?

But then again, you weren't you the day that you left.

That's how.

Useful Resources

Cynthia Chandler, *Animal-Assisted Therapy in Counseling*, (Fayetteville: Golden Waves of Books, 2011)

Wendy K. Williamson and Honora Rose Brentwood, *Two Bipolar Chicks Guide to Survival: Tips for Living with Bipolar Disorder*, (Brentwood: Post Hill Press, 2014)

Stephanie Taylor, *Animals That Heal: The Role of Service Dogs and Emotional Support Animals in Mental Health Treatment*, (Independently Published, 2018)

CHAPTER 3

Letting Go of Control (First Key)

It's not the load that breaks you down.
It's the way you carry it.
—Lena Horne

ACCORDING TO THE OXFORD Languages Dictionary the definition of *control* is "the power to influence or direct people's behavior or the course of events". No matter what you think or how hard you try, you can't actually control another person's behavior or actions. That person always has a choice to either follow your instructions or requests or to not.

I know what you are thinking! "If I whoop that bottom, they will do what I want." Is that true? Or do you find yourself scolding your child for similar actions over and over? I think scolding or spanking really just provides the parent with a release. Some children have a short memory, and once the memory of the incident fades, they'll take the same action again. So what have they learned? I find that natural consequences work a lot better. They allow the child to learn from their actions versus you telling them how wrong they are.

Typically, the tighter you hold on, the more they fight to get loose. It's like a dance with two people who don't like each other. Notice I didn't say they don't love each other. It is understandable to love your child and not like them at the same time due to their behavior. There were times when I thought: *How could she treat me this way when I am doing everything I can for her? I am trying to help her, not myself. If she doesn't change, she is going to make herself struggle.* The thing is, ultimately, that is her choice. She can choose to straighten up and fly right, as they say, or not. It is quite painful to witness, but you must let go.

It's like when you teach them to ride a bike. They start out with training wheels on the bike, and initially you are still holding the handlebars or the seat to keep them from falling. Then, at some point, once they realize that the training wheels will help them, you let go. Eventually you take the training wheels off, which means you go back to holding the handlebars or seat while they learn to balance the bike themselves. When you and your child feel confident enough, you let go so they can ride the bike on their own. You've got to believe that letting go is not giving up!

I've found that it is hard for a teenager to actually learn and understand what it takes for them to take care of themselves while living at home. But they will never learn these lessons if you don't relax that hold and let them try. Sure! There will be mistakes. That's how we all learned to be self-sufficient.

Of course, I am not saying that you should put your teenager out of the house. I am saying that when it is traditionally the time for them to launch after graduating high school, find a way to support their launch. This may look different for your child with mental health challenges. If they can't live on campus at a four-year college, maybe they can live with a roommate and attend community college, or maybe they take a gap year and participate in some type of residential community service program, or maybe they get a job and support themselves and their household. However it looks in your situation, the key is for you to *let go*. Trust that what you have poured into your child is in there. There isn't a hole for the information, lessons, and wisdom to leak out of.

Even though they may have resisted your rules and routines, that information is in there. You'll be surprised when they call on that information.

Since you can't control your child's behavior, consider how you can exercise control over your responses to your child. As I explored the issue of when and how to let go, I discovered that these issues are perplexing for many parents of children with mental health challenges.

Getting the correct mental illness diagnosis can be difficult. The medical community continues to research and develop different approaches and methodologies regarding mental illness. Age does play a factor in diagnoses. Bipolar disorder diagnosis typically occurs during latter teenage and young adult years. In talking to other parents, I learned that bipolar disorder has appeared in kids as young as those in kindergarten; however, it was frequently misdiagnosed as ADHD. Who knows? Either diagnosis could be right. There are certainly some similarities in symptoms.

Some diagnosticians claim bipolar disorder is over diagnosed. Others say it is not diagnosed early enough to give educators, parents, and clinicians a chance to teach coping strategies before letting go.

What Does Bipolar Disorder Look Like in Young Children?

In kids, some of the behaviors attributed to bipolar disorder may be more commonly recognized as ADHD. However, these behaviors may well be typical for young children. Diagnosis is certainly an issue. Is it one best left alone until children get older? Many experts agree.

Here's another problem: medications traditionally used to treat ADHD and bipolar disorder are often stimulants. These can be a trigger for mania in young children with bipolar disorder.

In kids, changes from high to low occur much more quickly. In adults, manic and depressive periods could be weeks, months, or even years apart. In young children they might happen in a single day. Highs and lows look different in children than they do in adolescents and adults.

How Can I Best Help My Child?

We all want to teach our kids social and job skills that will help them make their way in the world. If you are the parent of a child with a mental illness, you want to help them develop coping strategies for dealing with their condition.

There are many things you can do to help your child and keep them well. Other parents have offered these suggestions:

- When you consider letting go, medication can be a major concern. It is an absolute must that those on medication take the medication they need as prescribed. Thanks to modern technology, there is no shortage of reminder devices available, including timers, pill boxes, smartphone alarms, or notes. Pick the one that works best and develop a routine. If your child needs to take medication at school, talk to the principal or school nurse about protocol.

- Many medications used for mental illness may have side effects. It is important to be aware of the possible side effects medications like mood stabilizers, antipsychotic medications, and antidepressants may have. Many medications were tested on adults, not children. Some kids are more prone to side effects. These may include weight changes and fluctuations in blood sugar and cholesterol. There may even be an increased risk of suicide. Discuss medications and their side effects with your child's doctor. Keep a log.

- Keep a line of communication open with the school. Kids with mental illnesses may need special accommodations at school. They may need extra breaks or less homework during difficult times. Work out an agreement with your child's teachers, their school counselor, or the school principal. Often kids of any age need an advocate.

- A positive learning environment is important. In some cases, your child may need to be homeschooled—at least for a while.

- Routines are critical. Children with mental illnesses need a daily schedule. Sometimes they need help with or monitoring of getting up, maintaining daily hygiene, eating meals, exercising, doing homework, and going to bed on time.

- Part of letting go may be family therapy. Kids with mental illnesses can be disruptive to the whole family. Your marriage, other children, and work life can experience stress.

- Letting go by its very nature adds stress and upsets established routines. It may feel like one step forward and two steps back. The end goal may be a good one, but getting there may be painful.

- Letting go must occur in gradual steps. You cannot just cut the cord and say, "There you go, little bird. Fly away."

- Always have a plan B. If the loosening of control doesn't work, what's the next step?

- Constant communication is the key to making the letting-go process work.

Teenagers with Mental Illnesses

In older teenagers, symptoms and treatments of mental illness are like those seen in adults. But having a teenager with this condition presents unique problems.

As they get older, teenagers might be resentful if they feel that you're imposing treatment on them.

Encourage them to be part of the conversation. Talk frankly—along with your child's doctor or therapist—about treatment options. Try not to develop an adversarial relationship with your child over their treatment or medication. Approach it from the perspective that this is a family issue and mutual support is vital.

As with adults, it's key that teenagers with bipolar disorder avoid alcohol and drugs. These illegal substances can interact with prescribed medications, producing disastrous results.

All teens are at risk of developing substance abuse issues. For teens with bipolar disorder, the risk is significantly higher than it is for their peers.

I cannot stress enough the importance of routines and natural consequences. Kids need to have age-appropriate routines, responsibilities, and rules. Sleeping, getting up, maintaining personal hygiene, and performing household chores are important parts of being a family member.

Every family has expectations of its members. These should be appropriate for the child's age and ability.

Dr. Robert Myers, a clinical child and adolescent psychologist, outlines age-appropriate chores for kids in his article, "The Ultimate List of Age-Appropriate Chores."

He points out that two- and three-year-olds can complete chores like putting toys away, helping make their bed, and assisting with room tidying and pet care.

Preschoolers learn to complete tasks by copying adults and older siblings. They can dry mop floors, make their beds, clear the table, sort magazines, water plants, sort laundry, and shelve books with help.

School-aged children, ages six through nine, can do these tasks unsupervised as well as complete tasks including dusting, stacking and emptying the dishwasher, helping bring in groceries, setting the table, and folding laundry.

Older children can run the dishwasher, the washer, the dryer, and the vacuum cleaner, as well as care for pets. For children who suffer from mental illness, adjustments may need to be made.

However, all children who are part of the family unit should have realistic household responsibilities.

Download Dr. Meyers's list of age-appropriate chores here: https://childdevelopmentinfo.com/chores/the-ultimate-list-of-age-appropriate-chores/#gs.kuzxe0. Adapt it to suit your child's capabilities.

It's also important to maintain regular routines around sleep and wake times and to develop effective coping strategies for avoiding stress. It is a major trigger for mood disorders for all children.

Talk to your child's teachers. In some cases, you may need to take your child out of school for a while. Constant open communication with the school is vital. The educators need to know what is going on with your child in order to offer support. As a parent or caregiver, you can do a lot to help schools deal with students who have mental illnesses. You will be amazed at what parents and educators working together have accomplished. Here are some examples suggested by proactive parents:

- The first step is awareness. Staff and students need to be educated about mental health. They need help in recognizing the signs and knowing where to go for help and how they may help others.

- Keep the school informed about mental health issues and changes in symptoms and needs.

- Offer resources for mental health training. Educators need to know and understand basic mental health. This includes educating staff and students about the signs and symptoms of mental illness. Many parents host mental health evenings where they present an overview and answer questions from staff and parents.

- Advocate for a school open-door policy where kids feel safe and comfortable approaching staff. Even if staff does not feel qualified to deal with mental health issues, the willingness to listen and help find resources goes a long way.

- Encourage the school to have a "safe space" where students can talk to a counselor or volunteer.

- Promote good physical health. Students who eat nutritious foods, get adequate exercise, and receive at least eight hours of sleep are better able to handle mental challenges.

- Nurture social activities at school. These give students a chance to get outside themselves and see that they are more like others. Staff members are grateful for parental assistance in encouraging students to participate in a broad range of interactive opportunities during school. There may be opportunities to volunteer to help monitor and facilitate social activities during school hours.

- Encourage staff to build mental health into the curriculum. It can be integrated into literature, history, and health.

- Help organize a World Mental Health Day.

- Invite speakers from charities like Lee Thompson Young Foundation to share what they do to promote mental health education and support parents.

- Have a Wellness Week. Invite presenters to demonstrate tai chi, meditation, yoga, kickboxing, arts, crafts, hobbies, language learning, or ethnic cooking. Approach parents, teachers, and community members to help.

Consider family therapy. Having a child with a mental illness can be disruptive to the whole family. Your other children may not understand what's going on with their sibling. They may be resentful of all the attention their sibling is getting. Going to family therapy can help family members recognize and deal with these issues. Check out the information on family therapy in Chapter 8.

In-home therapy is part of mental health services for children and adults who suffer from severe mental health challenges. Also known as intensive in-home treatment, the program provides in-home mental health services for children and their families or caregivers. It was originally used with children at risk of out-of-home placements because of their extreme social, emotional, or behavioral challenges.

Intensive home therapy aims to keep children and their families together. The program provides individual and family counseling, as the name suggests, in the home or community. The goal is to help stabilize and decrease the youth's disruptive behaviors.

Fortunately, Nya's school was very flexible while we were going through in-home therapy. They knew her heart. They could have easily expelled her because she missed so many days, but they did not.

One of a caregiver's least appealing but most effective parenting strategies is tough love.

What is Tough Love?

Tough love forces us to take responsibility for our actions; it can literally save lives when it comes to those suffering from addiction issues or mental health problems. Tough love can also help us with simple daily tasks that we just don't feel like doing. When your mom tells you she isn't letting you go out for the night with your friends until you clean your room and finish your homework, that is tough love!

Tough love involves promoting a person's welfare. This is especially vital in situations involving mental health, addiction, or other challenging behaviors in your child, partner, sibling, or parent.

Tough love includes enforcing boundaries and requiring a person to take responsibility for their actions.

Tough Love Examples

Tough love involves strict discipline and communicating clearly defined obligations or requirements. This is done not to gain control but out of care for that individual—their safety and well-being. An example of tough love could be withholding a reward for getting a B in math because the desired grade was not achieved. Another example could be consequences for not doing chores or missing curfew.

Tough Love Advantages

When used properly and in a positive tone, practicing tough love makes relationships positive and consistent. If X...then Y...

However, if tough love is being used to manipulate, control, or coerce the individual, then it can become abusive.

Tough love guidelines and parameters should be discussed in family therapy. It should not be used for frivolous things like what to wear or whether to get a haircut.

If the situation is not serious or harmful, discussing the issue or letting your child make their own choice may be appropriate. Tough love should enhance relationships, not harm them. With tough love, behaviors and consequences are clearly, calmly, and quietly outlined at a time that is neither a high nor a low. If these discussions occur at bad times, relationships can deteriorate.

What are alternatives to tough love? Permissiveness, a laissez-faire attitude, babying, indulgence, pampering, overindulgence, coddling, mollycoddling, and ignoring bad behavior all have their consequences.

Why Use Tough Love with a Bipolar Situation?

Bipolar disorder need not be a barrier to healthy relationships, whether it is with a partner, a child, a sibling, or an aging parent.

Symptoms of bipolar disorder—not the condition itself—are often the cause of relationship problems.

There are many ways to treat bipolar disorder. A combination of medication and psychotherapy or alternative approaches may successfully reduce symptoms. However, behaviors and consequences often require a structured, consistent approach. Tough love offers such an approach. Yes, it is hard work. You feel mean as a parent. Others may judge you harshly. That is why it is important to discuss this in family therapy and with the life management team.

With the right treatment plan, those with bipolar disorder may have long periods when their mood is stable. They may experience mild symptoms that are unlikely to significantly affect their relationships.

Tough Love Tips

It's often pretty rough trying to cope with a manic-depressive loved one. You want desperately to help them, but sometimes the usual notions of what it means to help someone backfire. In fact, they are quite likely to backfire. Take it from someone who has been on both the receiving and the delivering end of tough love. It works. I did not say it was fun!

- Never forget that your loved one's illness is not your problem—nor is it your fault. Don't take it personally (see Chapter 4).

- Be firm and calm. Don't buy into the drama.

- Refuse to take any abuse. Walk away.

- Don't abandon if it's a safety issue. Be there as a safety net. Be a sounding board.

- Your presence lets your loved one know that it's okay to be angry at the disorder, but it is not okay to take that anger out on others.

- Be resilient to the "poor me" whine.

- Hard truths and painful honesty are part of tough love.

- Know that you may be a testing ground. Your loved one may be attempting to get a handle on how to exist as this newly diagnosed person.

- Be open and honest in a positive way.

- Acknowledge the person's emotions and then give them breathing room.

- Be sensitive to depression and grief involved in bipolar disorder.

- Try to empathize but don't presume you know what your loved one is going through.

- Set clear boundaries about behaviors that are not acceptable. Make the consequences absolutely clear.

Parents' and Partners' Dilemma

Here are some statements that I've made myself or heard from others over the years. I am sharing these statements, so you know that you are not alone:

> "The hard thing is, you try to help them, but you're still the bad one."

"Talk to yourself like you would to someone you love."

"My wife is in the middle of a manic episode. Her sister is insisting on 'tough love.' This means refusing to engage her unless she accepts her illness and resumes her full medication. If I don't, her sister says I am 'enabling' her behavior. Thus, she will see no need to change."

"Hospitalization seems to be the only way to get her to take her meds. She reverts as soon as her treatment team lets her come home."

"I have been continuing my 'tough love.' I minimize communication when she is hostile to me. She accuses me of abandoning her."

"I feel mean, torn, and abused. Tough love is wearing me out."

"I'm not telling you it is going to be easy. But I am telling you it is going to be worth it."

"Tough love does not mean being mean. It's called tough love because accepting the impossibility of changing someone else's behavior is tough to do."

"There is nothing wrong with setting clear boundaries. That's all tough love is."

POEM: MY JOB AS A MOM

One of my jobs is protecting you from harm,
which includes protecting you from yourself.
It doesn't seem like I'm doing a good job,
but I can say I'm doing the best I can.
But man,
when your self-harm appears,
it hurts me to my core,
because it is evidence of the struggle you feel.
When you were younger, you'd say, "Mom, the struggle is real."
I didn't get it then,
but now I do.
I just hope you choose *you*.
I know it's hard,
but you are worthy
of love,
success,
peace,
abundance.
You can choose to do better,
not because I say so,
but for yourself.
I pray that you will use the tools
you learn in therapy
to pause,
take a breath,
and choose wisely.
I hope you choose *you*
as you fall and get back up.

I'll be here to lend a helping hand
along with your dad,
but you have to accept the help.
Learn from your mistakes
and choose *you*
over the impulses that you feel,
because those impulses can steal
your hopes and dreams away, and
you deserve better.
You are beautiful.
You are strong,
gifted, and talented.
You are a blessing to us
and the children and the animals that you help.
I pray you choose *you*.

Useful Resources

Chelsea Lowe and Bruce M. Cohen, *Living with Someone Who's Living with Bipolar Disorder,* (San Francisco: Jossey Bass, 2010)

Paul T. T. Mason and Randi Kreger, *Stop Walking on Eggshells,* (New York: New Harbinger Publications, 2010)

James Dobson, *Love Must Be Tough,* (Nashville: W Pub Group, 1996)

Robert Meyers, (2019, October 14). "The Ultimate List of Age-Appropriate Chores." October 14, 2019, https://childdevelopmentinfo.com

Susan Rice, *Tough Love: My Story of the Things Worth Fighting For,* (New York: Simon & Schuster, 2019)

CHAPTER 4
Don't Take It Personally (Second Key)

Caregiving often calls us to lean into love we
didn't know possible.
—Tia Walker

THIS IS A VERY challenging lesson to learn. Have you ever felt attacked by your child or your loved one who has a mental illness? I know that I have. Mental health professionals will tell you that the things that your child says to you when they are upset or in a crisis should be treated like garbage. They suggest thinking of it as garbage that doesn't mean anything.

When you're in the moment, and you see that look in their eyes, and you know they're 100 percent serious, it seems like they know exactly what they're saying and that they mean every word of it.

In my experience, the words and the tone being used were personal for sure and directed at me. It seemed like my daughter was digging for words that she felt would be the most hurtful. The more I responded, the more hurtful her words became. It was like a dance that you don't want to be in.

I've mentioned previously doing this dance. It was as though anything I said was agitating and would lead to her ratcheting up her comments to be more and more aggressive.

Eventually I had to learn to change my responses and focus on myself instead of on what she was saying. I learned to leave the room to calm the situation or to at least protect myself in terms of my feelings. Leaving kept me from joining her on that negative level.

I would leave the room because I knew that she couldn't argue with herself. I felt like, *Well, if I'm not in the room, she's not going to keep arguing. There will be nobody there for her to direct her comments toward.*

That worked a couple of times. However, in the calm times, when we would be processing a particular episode with her psychiatrist, my daughter would say that it made her feel worse when I left. It was almost like a feeling of abandonment. Obviously, it was not my intention for her to feel abandoned. I was trying to leave that situation, not leave her, but that's how she perceived it.

The suggestion was made that I would announce that I was leaving. This would potentially help take the sting off of it. I would announce that I was using my own coping mechanism, and that would keep her from taking it personally. She would know that my action was meant as a coping mechanism intended to keep my emotions calm and to model what to do when you're upset. This way, she might not think that I was trying to leave her.

Then I tried that. I would announce it. And sometimes when I would leave, she would follow me in a rage. This then made it more personal, and I felt more attacked. Let me state that I was never physically attacked, but I felt attacked emotionally. I felt attacked, disrespected, and not loved.

At some point, leaving the room didn't necessarily work. Then I would leave the house for fifteen or twenty minutes until things calmed down.

From my perspective, I felt that when Nya was upset and experiencing a crisis, she did have feelings of hate toward me. In those moments, she was not able to recall anything that I'd done for her that was good. She felt like she didn't need me and was willing to do anything to get away from me at that time.

All of the time that you've spent on their behalf, fighting their issues and advocating for them, counts for nothing. All the money that you've spent, the emotions you've felt, and the love that you've poured into them—none of that is recognized when they're in a crisis.

So let me just set that expectation if you have not experienced it. What I learned to do is let her get those emotions out.

I might say something like, "I understand that you're upset right now," or "It doesn't seem like we're able to find a solution at this moment," or "I hear what you're saying."

Then I would reflect back to my daughter and say, "When you are calm, I would like to help you resolve this situation. When you're calm, maybe you can let me know what support looks like for you. But right now, when we're in this heightened state of emotion, I feel like it's difficult to figure out a solution or what might work or what the options are. So I am going to go and maybe take some deep breaths and take a break. Whenever you're ready to work through the situation and your thoughts, you can let me know. Choose a time that's good for both of us. Remember, when I'm cooking or working, my attention is elsewhere. That's not really a good time. When both of us have some time, and we're both calm, we can work through this situation in a positive way. I'd be happy to do that. But I'm going to leave now."

I would do that. Initially it was quite unnerving for my daughter. I would leave her room or whatever room we were talking in. I could hear her, still screaming or hitting the bed, letting her frustration out. I wouldn't go back. Sometimes we make the mistake of going back to see if they're okay or to say, "Hey! That's not necessary!" and that kind of thing. These types of attempts only stir things up, even though our intention is to help resolve the situation. These types of actions would cause my daughter to get agitated again. I would not go back unless I heard something that was concerning, like something breaking or her throwing something.

More often than not, the approach of announcing that I was leaving and letting her know that I would be there for her once the situation had calmed worked.

After about five minutes or so, I would not hear any more screaming or hitting of things. At some point, she would either text me or come find me to have a productive conversation about whatever it was that had triggered her in the first place.

The conversation was not always productive. It didn't necessarily always result in Nya getting what it was that she was looking for or an absolute resolution to whatever it was that had made her so upset.

But because the conversation was calm and we could talk through what it was that had triggered her and what it was she was expecting versus what I was expecting, we could come to some type of solution or find a way forward in a collaborative manner.

You might think of it as similar to how you would approach a conflict at work. With a colleague, you would provide a safe space, let some time pass by, and then revisit the issue to find a way forward that is mutually beneficial to both parties. That same approach can be effective at home with your children.

Keep in mind that things may change as your child gets older. Children develop and mature over time. As a result of that growth, you may need to adjust your approach to resolve conflicts. There might be a particular tactic that you used when they were younger, let's say ten or younger, and then when they transition into the preteen or teenage years, you may need to adjust that tactic. As parents, we should also be aware of possible manipulation from our children. Sometimes they know our "weak" spots and can use just the right language to get what they want, even though we know they need something different from us.

In my experience, in the cases that I have come across in terms of emotional disorders such as bipolar, like with my daughter and my brother, most of these people are extremely intelligent. Often they know what words or actions will trigger you. If you let them trigger you, you've taken the bait. We have a choice, right? If you let them trigger you, then you are playing into their hands. That's what they want. They are seeking that engagement and the ongoing banter. Then they can blame things on you instead of taking responsibility.

You have to find a way to take the high road when they are taking the low road. You have to put on your big girl panties or your big boy pants, and you have to be a mature adult when dealing with these situations. Also, have the courage to reach out and get help and support for yourself as the parent.

Parents I have talked to over the years say that it's one of the toughest things they have to deal with. That's why I included a section on tough love in the previous chapter.

As I mentioned earlier, we had therapists for my daughter: a talk therapist and a psychiatrist. Then I had to get my own therapist to help with parenting. We also had intensive in-home therapy at one point when my daughter was going through a crisis, and that was for the family.

I think there is a misconception out there that the person with the mental illness or emotional challenges is the patient, and thus you need to do all these things for them. But their illness impacts the entire family. Everyone in the home is impacted. Everything you are doing for them is also for yourself and for everyone else in the family.

I am an advocate for family therapy. It is very helpful. That would involve both parents and any siblings who are in the home. If there are grandparents or other relatives in the home or close by, they should be involved in the family therapy if possible. Check out my family therapy advice in Chapter 8.

If all household members are not involved in family therapy, what happens is that, unintentionally, there is a disjointed approach to supporting the person with the illness. You may be undoing some of the coping plans that they are going over with their therapist if you're saying something different, not knowing that you're saying something different. Or you might be reinforcing "bad behaviors," not knowing that you're doing that. If you're informed because of the therapy, then you know that the whole village or family that lives in your home can better support the person with the illness and help them to develop. In the end, that person is responsible for their actions.

They have an illness that can make it challenging to make what we would consider to be the right choices and take the right actions and say the right things. They have an illness that makes that challenging, but that person has to accept that illness and learn how to manage it.

That illness is an explanation of their behavior. It is not an excuse for bad behavior. An illness does not make misbehavior okay. It explains why it happened. As family members, along with the mental health professionals, we have to work with them to help them to be able to accept it and then figure out how to manage it in a way that resonates with them.

Unfortunately, there is no one-size-fits-all solution, but there are people who are successfully managing their mood disorders. You just have to figure out what works for you, and help your child figure out what resonates with them and what's going to make this a plan of least resistance.

You must remember it is an actual illness, so no matter what it is that they're saying to you, it is being filtered through that illness. You should keep telling yourself not to take it personally, step back, and do what you need to do for your own self-care so that when they calm down, you can show up as your best self, as their parent to help them take the next right step forward.

There is a stigma attached to those with mental illnesses. Unfortunately, the frustration these people feel about other people's expectations of them often gets misdirected to the very people who care and are trying to be understanding and supportive. Sometimes the parents or caregivers get emotionally attacked by the person and the public, but as parents we continue on because our love is unconditional.

In the following chapter, we'll talk more about the stigma of living with and caring for a person with a mental illness.

It's very hard not to take hurtful remarks personally. It's even harder when you are the caregiver who has given up countless hours to make life better for your child and your family. Believe me! I feel your pain. You deserve better. Remember, it's not your son or daughter, your sibling, or your parent lashing out at you. It's the disease talking.

POEM: DON'T TAKE IT PERSONALLY

You sent her here,
but she's always gone.
My touch doesn't comfort her.
My nurturing is repelling to her.
Now I feel alone.

It's like love is not welcomed by her.
She is constantly withdrawing
and pushing us away.
Yet I still try to look forward to another day.

Don't take it personally, they say.
Okay.

Easier said than done,
but I know it is necessary.

And when I'm able to do it,
I feel like I've won.

At least for that day.

Then I move forward
one step at a time.

Useful Resources

Rosalie Greenburg, *Bipolar Kids: Helping Your Child Find Calm in the Mood Storm*, (Lebanon: Da Capo Lifelong Books, 2008)

Demitri Papolos and Janice Papolos, *The Bipolar Child*, (New York: Harmony, 2007)

Heather Rose, *Bipolar Child: Bipolar Survival Guide for Children*, (Newark: Speedy Publishing LLC, 2015)

Janet Wozniak and Mary Ann McDonnell, *Positive Parenting for Bipolar Kids*, (New York: Bantam, 2009)

CHAPTER 5

From Grief to Healing (Third Key)

Grief only exists where love lived first.
—Franchesca Cox

YOU MAY BE WONDERING why I am addressing grief when this book is about surviving the mental health tank and parenting a child with a mental illness.

If the first reaction you had to your child's diagnosis was grief, then you're normal! I had the same reaction. Even though I felt relief that someone had finally put a name to what my child was suffering from, I also felt grief because mental illness was the label.

Most of us who are parenting a child or caregiving for our loved one with a mental illness have grief because we experience loss. Whenever that person has a setback, an episode, something disappointing, or something that you thought they were going to be able to do and it's just not panning out, that is a loss.

If you have other children, it is natural to subconsciously or consciously compare your children. The one who has the mental illness is struggling in some aspect of their life. You feel a loss.

I think this is why, as parents, we want to fill the gap. We want to fix the problem. We want to encourage them to do better. Sometimes they're already doing the best that they can. You know the saying: each day is not promised. Each day you don't know what you're going to get. Unfortunately, that's the nature of a mood disorder and particularly bipolar disorder. I'm speaking from my experience of raising a daughter with bipolar disorder.

You don't know if it's going to be a good day or a bad day. So when you have the good days, it's like you're just holding your breath, waiting for the other shoe to drop, for the next bomb to go off in your child's life and in your life and your household.

That's a loss of peace. There is a loss of freedom. You're bracing yourself for this journey. I've had mental health professionals tell me to hold on for the ride. It is typically a roller coaster, and it feels like it's never-ending. Just hold on because eventually it gets better.

When the experts say "eventually," they can't actually give you a time frame. So you don't know how long you're supposed to be holding on. Some of the roller coaster drops are excruciating. It can feel like you're actually upside-down, or you've been thrust up out of your seat and you're holding on for dear life.

When there is an episode or a crisis with your loved one, you are conscious. You know that the situation is temporary, and at some point, you're going to get through this. You tell yourself, "Hey! I've gotten through this before, and I can get through it again."

But, in that moment, you don't know when it's going to end. One minute feels like ten minutes. Each time you feel like you are not sure this is actually going to get better.

That is a loss. You know that evening or that morning or that day or that night—when the episode and crisis occurs, whether it's a short time period or over multiple days—you've lost that time. You've lost a sense of peace and harmony, and you don't know when you're going to get it back. That's grief.

I found myself feeling sad for myself and my daughter. Because of her illness, she had been robbed of certain experiences, certain joys in her life. And in turn, I had been robbed because she wasn't able to experience those things, and I wasn't able to experience those things through her. I think one of the things I've learned is to accept that grief and let it out. It's okay to be sad. One of the things that I would always tell myself is, "Hey! It could be worse."

On the other hand…I know it could be worse, but that doesn't diminish the pain and the struggle that my child is going through and what I'm going through as a parent. It doesn't make it any easier for me just because I know that some people have it worse. The pain and the level of pain and struggle that we're experiencing is real. And it's okay to be sad about that. You don't want to be debilitated by that sadness. You want to keep putting one foot in front of the other and do the best that you can. But it is certainly expected and okay to feel sad. You need someone who you can talk to and express your disappointment to. Maybe you can even discuss your own depression about the situation that is occurring with your child, due to these mental health challenges. Expressing it can provide a sense of relief to you, and that is what I experienced.

I knew that I needed certain things at certain times. If I had not let out that frustration, that grief, that sadness, it was going to make me sick. I remember having times when I felt like I was nauseous. I just had so much going on, and I was trying so hard to handle everything that I felt sick.

This is when I leaned on my tribe. It is good to know your tribe and who you can turn to for what. There are certain people who I call to vent to. If I need someone to boost me up, encourage me, and tell me I'm a champion and that they believe I can do this, I call someone different. There were times when I'd had enough, and I had to get away. My husband always understood this, and he was there to handle things at home while I was gone. I know people have different levels of resources, so there may be different things you are able to do for self-care.

With my trusted others, we talk about what is going on, and we are intentional about self-care. There are creative things that you can do for self-care that will help you. These things will actually build up your resilience so that when it is a tough time, a challenging time, a crisis, an episode, you are better equipped to handle it.

You can build up your resilience through your own intentional self-care routines. This is so important that my final chapter is dedicated to self-care processes.

You have to name the grief and deal with it. In my experience, the really tough times began when my daughter was in middle school and continued through her high school years. There were things that she liked to do and that we encouraged her to do as parents. There were talents we saw in her that she didn't necessarily see in herself. My daughter is a natural swimmer, but she also loved basketball. She chose to pursue basketball instead of swimming because the seasons overlapped. She swam in elementary school and then somewhere around middle school, maybe seventh grade, she decided she couldn't do both with the overlapping seasons. She chose basketball. As her parents, we were thinking, *No! You're a natural swimmer.*

It's her journey. So, as her parent, I'm here to support her on her journey. I said, "Okay! That's what you want to do? Then that's what we'll do."

So we did basketball. The thing about basketball and mood disorders, which can be kind of challenging, is that you're a member of a team. You're a member of a team as a swimmer too, but basketball is much more integrated. It's a team sport. Working as a team is the whole point. If you're having an off day, you let your team down. Either you show up and can't focus, or you don't show up and leave the team missing a player. Your team could begin to resent your highs and lows. Do you explain what's happening to your team and risk the stigma? Are you even able to articulate it in a way that your team members can understand?

When you're not feeling well and experiencing mood swings, you're not just impacting yourself. If you're in a swimming event, you are also impacting the team; however, they may be able to substitute another swimmer more easily than they could with a starting basketball player. It can be challenging to manage the team dynamic. When you don't show up, or when you're not engaged in basketball practice and then you come off the bench instead of starting, then you have to manage your emotions because now you're disappointed in yourself, and you're not contributing at your best level for the team. Playing a sport is a lot to manage whether or not you have a mental illness. I've covered some of the challenges of playing a sport from my perspective as a parent. On the positive side, the physical fitness and social skills developed can be very helpful in managing a mental illness.

Looking at this as a parent and experiencing this while my daughter was going through it felt like a loss because I wanted the experience of playing a team sport to be simple and joyful for her.

I wanted her to be able to enjoy that time as a teenager, to thrive and learn from being part of a team. I feel she did learn from being part of a team. But the stakes were so high that I felt like we were walking on eggshells. The stress was high. The heightened stress level set off bipolar episodes. It was a vicious cycle.

I felt at some point that the whole team dynamic became too much. There were other players on Nya's team with mental health challenges, so their emotions were up and down too. Their mood swings impacted Nya, which felt like a loss.

There were good times and exciting times. As a parent, you support your children. I enjoyed going to the games and cheering, especially when Nya was scoring buckets! It was like, "Yes! She is doing it, and we are doing it!"

Then, all of a sudden, we couldn't do it. Nya decided that she wasn't going to play basketball anymore. She was feeling depressed and unmotivated. That was a loss.

There's grief on this journey whether you realize it or not. So you need to do something to allow that grief and sadness to come out. Address that sadness and then move on.

There may be "normal," expected activities that your child is not able to participate in. In high school, typically you go to the homecoming dance and to the prom. You may hang out with your friends, or you may be dating. But when you have a mood disorder, sometimes those things don't come as easily. And the way that I've heard my daughter explain it, based on my memory, is that she would rather not ask someone to hang out and risk them saying that they're not available. This is because she doesn't know if they're really not available or if they just don't want to hang out with her. So she would just rather be alone and not ask.

I've witnessed this and encouraged her, but she was uncomfortable. She did not want to invite anyone to do anything. I had to remind myself that it was her journey.

When she was a younger child, I arranged playdates and outings. They were fine. I don't remember any negative incidents. But certainly, as a teenager, it had to be her choice. There were times when she would be invited to go somewhere. Typically, she would go, and she would enjoy herself, or she would at least say that she had enjoyed herself.

But in her later teen years, she admitted that she felt she had some social anxiety. When she did hang out with her friends, I'm not sure that they could tell that she was happy to be there or that she was enjoying herself because she was experiencing anxiety the entire time. Maybe she wasn't saying anything. Maybe she wasn't interacting. Maybe she was on her phone. But it was not because she didn't want to be there; it was because of social anxiety.

Again, that is a loss of what we consider to be a "normal experience." I'm sharing this information so that you have some examples. This may or may not be happening in your situation. But I think it's helpful for you to know that this can happen. Who's to say what is normal, right? Here's my point: if you're trying to compare your child's experience to your experience growing up, and you didn't have those types of challenges, then nine times out of ten, their experience is very different from what you experienced as a teenager and what you expect their experience to be. You naturally grieve the absence of the experiences in your formative years that you feel your child is missing out on. While your feelings are valid, remember it's not your journey.

Now let's address another type of grief: actual physical loss of a loved one. This could be through a death, like we experienced when we lost my brother, Lee, or Nya's great-grandmother. It might involve the loss of a beloved pet or a school friend who moves away. It might be a move to a new school, a new house, or a new community. It may involve family splits.

Kids with bipolar disorder need and crave routines. Disruptions cause stress. This, in turn, increases high and low episodes.

More research is needed regarding grief in those with bipolar disorder. Unsurprisingly, there is little information on how to process grief and what resources exist to offer practical support.

Grief counseling for those with bipolar disorder dealing with loss should be offered by someone with both training in grief counseling and a good knowledge of bipolar disorder. Standard bereavement options are, at best, hit or miss.

Grief and stress are individual triggers. Put them together and add disruptions in routines and feelings of abandonment, and you can see how loss can lead to a crisis time.

Because grief is a trigger, rapid cycling often occurs. This all occurs even in the presence of optimum medication intervention.

Beware of delayed grief. After my brother's death, Nya received counseling. She seemed to have processed Lee's death okay, until she began having behavioral issues at school. These behavioral issues began to spiral out of control. She returned to grief counseling. Loss of any kind can trigger a relapse.

I believe that bipolar disorder may cause delays in the grief process. In the midst of highs and lows, there is little space for grieving and little energy to devote to it. Grief and depression are not the same. They are both lows but require different approaches. In a state of manic high, those with bipolar disorder are out of touch with grief. Their focus is euphoria. Those good feelings distract from grief.

Some people may set grief aside for a period of time and have to play catch up later. Grieving is a necessary step to coming to terms with a loss. If this doesn't occur, we can be caught in hidden grief that acts as a mood trigger.

How can we grieve? Find ways to override the mood symptoms. Journaling may help to treasure the good memories. Nya is a writer, and I journal. We treasure items that Lee gave us prior to his death, and sometimes we talk about the good times we shared with Lee.

Grief needs space. You need time to become aware of your grief. Check in with your feelings. Come to terms with the fact your loved one is really gone. Identify the source of what you are feeling, and acknowledge the legitimacy of your feelings.

When depression sets in, take some time to manage your feelings. Connect with what you are feeling. Ask yourself, "How am I?" Don't curl up, roll over, and ignore any discomfort. Just focus on it. This is a good way to connect with reality.

There are ways to alleviate grief. Sit quietly. Look at old photos or a scrapbook or think of a pleasant memory. Read something that resonates with you. Listen to music. Write. Create. Go for a walk.

Maintain a "How am I?" journal to check in with yourself each day. Write as little or as much as you want.

Keep a memory box. Go through it regularly. Remind yourself of why you included each item. Add new items. You might be surprised at the emotions these things bring up.

Practice self-care. Wrap yourself up in a blanket or fuzzy sweater. Enjoy your favorite beverage. Acknowledge your sorrow and remember the good times.

Whether we are grieving for a person, a pet, a friend who has moved away, an unattained milestone, or the loss of an ability we once had, these feelings need a place to vent.

A large part of surviving grief over bipolar disorder is dealing with survivor's guilt.

Addressing Survivor's Guilt

You don't have to struggle in silence. You can be un-silent. You can live well with a mental health condition, as long as you open up to somebody about it, because it's really important you share your experience with people so that you can get the help that you need.

—Demi Lovato, *The Cut* interview (2017)

My brother died alone. The agony and stigma around bipolar disorder made his life unbearable. Initially I was consumed with guilt and self-blame. I was his sister. We were close. How could I have been so wrapped up in my life that I'd missed the signs? I worked through several sessions with a therapist to forgive my brother and myself.

The Lee Thompson Young Foundation provides an opportunity for me to help others as a result of surviving the loss of my brother. It provides a purpose greater than myself. During the early years, my daughters would volunteer with me at local health fairs to promote mental health education.

What Is Self-Blame?

Self-blame is a thought process through which an individual attributes the blame for a stressful event to themselves. This feeling of guilt is linked to their behaviors or feelings. Blame can be stressful. It can affect future success, as the person who blames themselves feels unworthy.

Self-blame is often a reaction to a stressful event, like Lee's death by suicide or Nya's diagnosis. In both cases, I felt responsible—like I should have done something to prevent these traumatic events.

Self-blame can—and frequently does—contribute to depression. Thanks to my family, friends, and therapists, I was able to adapt, but it was a slow process.

Self-blame is also associated with guilt and self-disgust. Because of these links, self-blame should be carefully monitored.

Through initiatives like my nonprofit, my speaking engagements, my social media posts, and my parent success course, I have been able to turn my guilt and self-blame into something positive and constructive.

Others have also turned negative feelings into positive outcomes. Emily runs a center where she is part of a facility that helps others who are trying to work their way through feelings of guilt and low self-esteem.

Like me, Brandon took to the speaker's circuit after his twenty-two-year-old daughter died of a deliberate medication overdose. Brandon quit his job as a defense attorney to reach out to parents of other children with bipolar disorder. "I wasn't there for Laura," he said quietly. "I want to raise awareness so no parent has to go through what my family endured." To date, he has taken his message to over ten thousand people.

Marissa has started a kids' help line, especially for youth with bipolar disorder who are feeling lonely, unloved, ignored, depressed, or suicidal. She is assisted by adults and youth who have been diagnosed with bipolar disorder or are living with a diagnosed family member.

Cindy has discovered that by helping others, she feels better about herself. Her helping projects have included volunteering on an alpaca farm, catering, reading to seniors, attending cooking classes for young moms, and gardening in small spaces.

A runner in high school, Alana took up marathon running to combat survivor's guilt after her friend was killed in the car she was driving. "Everyone said it wasn't my fault. In my head I knew this, but my heart refused to listen. So I laced up my runners and literally outran my demons." Now Alana teaches those who are battling depression, grief, or self-blame how to run for mental wellness.

"Don't allow blame to color your life," challenges life coach David Rogers. He urges his clients to accept responsibility for their actions. "Admit your mistake. Fix it and move on. Don't give others a chance to attach blame. Learn from your mistakes."

Leah teaches her clients to practice self-love. "When they come to me all riddled with self-blame and self-loathing, I urge them to park those feelings at the door. We work on their positive traits. Sadly, many of them can't remember their strengths, but they are quick to list their shortcomings. In my workshops, we focus on strengthening their weaknesses and supplementing the positive traits," she adds.

What do all these people have in common? They've all experienced self-blame, guilt, or self-loathing. Rather than wallowing in self-pity, they have taken life's lemons and made lemonade. But they haven't just healed themselves. They have taken what they have learned and used it to help others heal.

POEM: RECREATE

So now you know my feelings about the past,
and I am supposed to process, grieve, and move on,
but not too fast.

I am supposed to find a new way of being
without you here.

What I feel now is supposed to be my new "normal,"
although it isn't "normal" at all.

"It is what it is," they say, and I will do the best I can
to manage it all,
to find out who I am again.

I am supposed to recreate myself as my heart mends
and try to be whole and well again.

I know I am still a businesswoman, a wife, a mom, a daughter,
a cousin, a friend.

I am just not sure my heart will ever mend,
not completely,
and I think that is okay.

Remember, "It is what it is," as they say.

I'll always be your big sis, Mu.
No need to recreate that.

Useful Resources

Matt Duczeminski, *"How to Stop Self-Blaming and Start Forgiving Yourself."* December 1, 2021, https://www.lifehack. org

Peg Streep, *"Tackling Self-Blame and Self-Criticism."* January 10, 2018, https://www.psychologytoday.com

Anita Agers-Brooks, *Getting through What You Can't Get Over*, (Uhrichsville: Barbour Books, 2015)

Anne Corlett, *The Space between the Stars*, (New York: Berkley, 2017)

Ashley Davis Bush, *Transcending Loss*, (New York: Berkley, 1997)

Michael Newman, *Hope When Your Heart Breaks: Navigating Grief and Loss*, (St. Louis: Concordia, 2017)

Michael Pierce, *Loss: A Practical Guide for Coping with Loss*, (Carlsbad: Balboa Press, 2016)

Alan Wolfelt, *Too Much Loss: Coping with Grief Overload*, (Chicago: Companion Press, 2020)

CHAPTER 6

Manage Your Expectations (Fourth Key)

Never underestimate your problem or your ability
to deal with it.
—Robert H. Schuller

THIS IS HARD TO do, especially for us moms. Take a minute to think about what you want for your child. Do you want your children to exceed your achievements? How do you want their lives to be? I'm sure you desire for things to go smoothly and meet or even exceed your expectations. These are typical parent wishes. We want our kids to do better than we did. We want them to be successful and fulfilled.

Are you comparing your child with mental health challenges to other people's children and to your other children? It's okay if you are. It's only human nature. We want the best for our children, and we often say that we want them to have it better than we did.

So whatever it was that we went through, however we grew up, we want it to be easier for our children. However we define better, we want that for our children.

That is actually putting expectations on your child. It could be simple things, like how I expected for my daughter to blossom when she got to middle school and have friends and have meetups and sleepovers and possibly a boyfriend. Then, in high school, I expected her to want to hang out with her friends and go to school dances, homecoming, and the prom. I expected her to want to wear makeup, dress up, and drive. And I expected her to want to go to college, work, and be able to support herself. I expected her to be happy.

That was not necessarily the case. These were expectations of mine that didn't necessarily align with Nya's expectations of herself. She may not have been capable of achieving these expectations at the time, and she may not have been motivated.

Whatever it is that I defined as "normal" was not my daughter's experience. It was not Nya's experience. Honestly? I'm not sure if she would say that she had a good high school experience. Actually, she might say that she did because she has a tendency to detach herself from any challenging incidents or memories. She typically remembers only the things that she considers to be positive. I think this is part of her coping mechanism.

My point here is if you set what you deem to be "normal expectations," and your child is wired differently, then you're almost always in a state of disappointment. Whether you mean to or not, you are trying to somehow guide your child in the direction of your expectations and convince them to share the expectations that you have for them. This can be frustrating for the child and for you.

It doesn't matter if you don't directly say, "Hey, I think you should do this. Everybody does it. I want you to have this normal experience." You don't have to say that because your child feels it.

They feel it in the way you talk to them. You encourage some things and discourage other things. Your child just may not want to do that. They may not have the capacity to do those things that you want them to do.

As mentioned earlier, instead of asking her friends to hang out, Nya would rather not ask at all and isolate herself in her room. To her, that was less stressful.

What we think should be easy and enjoyable for our child may not necessarily be. So this is when listening comes into play. Listen to your children who are dealing with mental illnesses. Read their body language and their nonverbal cues when they're trying to explain things to you.

You can do things, particularly with younger children, to foster relationships and try to take that pressure off relationships that our children sometimes feel. But once they get to be older teenagers, it becomes awkward for them if you're calling their friends' parents to arrange gatherings. With the best of intentions, you can do more harm than good.

I chose not to call around on behalf of my teenage daughter. I would make offers to Nya. I would try to make it easy for her to hang out by letting her know that she could invite someone over, or I could take her to meet a friend. At least she knew that I was fine with it. It was one less thing that she would need to worry about.

Remember that not managing your expectations causes you to live in a constant state of disappointment. That is not a good feeling. That is a sad feeling. I want you to be aware of this potential pitfall, so you can avoid it.

When you have multiple children, I think it's hard not to compare them. I'm not saying that you would be talking about and comparing them in front of them. But, in your mind, you may be thinking about why it is easy for this one and not for that one.

That constant disappointment breeds more frustration with the situation and for the child. They can feel that. They may interpret it as their not being good enough, not measuring up.

This is the opposite of what you want. We want to be sure that we are encouraging our children to do whatever it is that works for them, however it works for them. We advocate on their behalf with the schools or with their employers when they begin to work. We should continually model that advocacy, so they can learn to advocate for themselves.

We let them know that it's okay to ask for accommodations, whatever those might be. If they are feeling anxiety when they go to school about having a large number of people around, they can ask the teacher or the principal for accommodations—whatever the process is at your child's school. The child can ask if there is a safe space where they can go when they're feeling anxious, instead of them wanting to stay home, not go to school at all, and not face people.

From my experience, once that safe space is created, it is very helpful to the student dealing with mental health challenges. It may be a small room, or it may be in the principal's office, somewhere where they are away from the crowd.

Once that safe space is created, then they have room to process that anxiety. Eventually, they can join the typical classroom again.

This may take some time, but you want your child to feel safe in their learning environment. It may not be that day, and it may not be the next day, but that is certainly what you want (as opposed to your child staying at home and not going to school at all due to anxiety or depression).

You, as a parent, can manage your expectations. You can take the cues from your child. You can figure out what it is that will work for them. You can decide what a positive expectation is for them. They can realize what their norm is. The sooner you do that, the better. Then you can embrace it. If you don't, you are fighting against it, which is not helpful.

If you can do this, instead of trying to fight this uphill battle to accomplish these things that you consider to be the norm, you will be able to step back and see the situation as it is, not as you would wish it to be.

We need to stop aiming for accomplishing what looks like success for our child through our eyes. Have you asked your child what success means through their eyes?

Obviously, you still want to guide your child's relationships. You want to help them avoid social gaffes that can destroy their already tenuous self-concept. You still want to be a positive force. If they're making a decision that you know may not lead to the best outcome, you want to ask some questions so they can think about it. You want them to make wise, thought-out decisions.

Kids who deal with mental illnesses don't always have age-appropriate decision-making skills.

You need to remember: your kids are not living their lives to meet your expectations. They are on their own journey.

Our job is to manage our expectations. It is our job to support our children in a healthy way that helps them move forward. But this path they are taking must be in a direction that resonates with them. How can we learn to manage our expectations?

Where Does the Journey Begin?
The answer may seem obvious. The journey begins with your child's diagnosis at a doctor's office or when you observe that there is a problem at home.

Bipolar diagnoses typically happen between ages fifteen and nineteen. The second most frequent age range is twenty to twenty-four. Some don't experience their first manic episode until they are over fifty.

Some first signs may occur much earlier but may not be diagnosed as bipolar disorder.

Possible Signs of Bipolar Disorder
These are often mislabeled as depression or a hormonal imbalance for years before the bipolar diagnosis. Symptoms often include any or all of the following:

- Sadness or hopelessness
- Irritability most of the time
- Lacking energy, listlessness, or lethargy
- Difficulty concentrating and remembering things
- Loss of interest in everyday activities
- Feelings of emptiness
- Low self-worth
- Guilt or despair
- Negative self-talk
- Pessimism about everything
- Self-doubt
- Self-defeat

Parental Concerns That Things Are Not Quite Right

One parent noted that when his child was very young, he knew there was something different about his child. "He was so full of energy that he never sat still." This behavior often leads to a misdiagnosis of ADHD.

Fearlessness is also an early sign. Parents reported: "He had no fear of anything or anyone." There is always the worry that they will "wander off with a stranger."

Another early sign is night terrors. "The first time it happened, I thought the house was on fire. I had never heard him scream like that. I never heard anyone scream like that in their sleep," a parent noted.

Many children later diagnosed as bipolar were very aggressive at a young age. A mother described her daughter's aggression thusly: "When the terrible twos occurred at our house, our daughter would call me names and use toys as weapons if she didn't get her way."

A father said of his child, "A look would come over his face. *This child is possessed,* I'd think."

A frustrated mom told me, "No one had to tell me there was something wrong with my child. I have three other kids. Of course I knew this wasn't normal behavior. And I resented the attitude that because I don't have a medical degree, I know nothing. Parents know their kids."

Aggressive, angry behavior seems to increase at school age. "When he attempted to kick his kindergarten teacher, I knew it was time to look for help," one parent said. "The school seemed to think I had permissive parenting flaws."

Treatment Options

Another parent reported that she began with her daughter's pediatrician "he was attentive but seemed unsure where to go. He suggested I put my child on a special diet that eliminated red dye, caffeine, and milk. I think he was secretly diagnosing her symptoms as ADHD. What did I care what he called it as long as it cured the behavior?"

One parent reported that her medical team suggested behavioral therapy. Next they suggested vitamin therapy because her son had high LED levels and some vitamin deficiencies. "They claimed it was why my son was so hyper. The vitamin therapy involved asking a six-year-old to swallow several horse pills."

Keep in mind that with every new ailment, there are a lot of trial-and-error experiments. Some fail.

Medications aren't really the only solution. Moreover, medication comes with its own problems. "In the early days," stated one parent, "it was our best option."

"If I had to write a guide for parents whose child had just been diagnosed with bipolar disorder at any age," said a parent, "I would tell them to trust their instincts. Parents know."

Another parent agreed: "If you think something is wrong with your child, you are probably right. Educators or doctors might discount your concerns. Don't let them dissuade you. There is *no test* for bipolar. First, they rule other stuff out. If it's not this or this, then it may be bipolar."

One of my main frustrations with mental illness is that there is no one-size treatment that fits all. It is a process of trial and error to get to a treatment approach that works for your child.

Is Bipolar Hereditary?

Again, this might seem as weird a question as, "Is bipolar contagious?"

Bipolar is frequently thought to be inherited. Recent research shows that genetics account for an estimated 80 percent of bipolar disorder cases.

What are the odds? Not as grim as you might think. If one of your parents has bipolar disorder, there's a one in ten chance that you will get it too. While it is not hereditary, if you have bipolar disorder, you were likely born with a predisposition for it.

So what does a predisposition mean? Mental illnesses sometimes run-in families; thus, if you have a family member with a mental illness, you may be somewhat more likely to develop a mental illness. On the other hand, you could experience a stressful life event that might trigger the onset of bipolar disorder or other mental illnesses.

How Can You Manage Your Expectations as the Parent of a Child with a Bipolar Diagnosis?

This is a bit of a tricky question. The onset of bipolar disorder typically occurs from the early to midtwenties. At that point, you no longer have legal authority over your child. Nevertheless, you're understandably concerned about how bipolar disorder may affect your child's life and their livelihood. While your child may push back, they need your support now more than ever. This is a turbulent time for them. They need as much "ordinary," "predicable," and "normal" as you can provide.

Adjusting Your Expectations

First, let's consider what is actually realistic. It's commendable to have a "can do" attitude, *but* are we espousing an unattainable ideal? Is that beyond the reach for many newly diagnosed adults or teens? This can be a tough age for all kids. Bipolar disorder adds an extra weight. I am not saying to set no expectations. Just be aware and adjust with empathy. Bipolar symptoms recur in up to 90 percent of those diagnosed with the disorder at any age.

Making the changes that bipolar disorder demands and making the necessary adaptations emotionally and behaviorally takes time and maturity that many kids this age don't have. This is where you can help.

Try not to fixate on goals, milestones, and expectations. Concentrate on your child's feelings. This will help you and your child get a handle on their bipolar disorder and what it actually looks and acts like for your child.

You need experience living with the disorder. This is your new reality. It's completely different from your perceived reality. Focus on the details for now.

Helpful Suggestions for Parenting a Child with a Mental Illness

Parenting a child with a mental illness *is* stressful and frustrating. Let's not minimize this.

Park the guilt outside. You are not to blame for your child's mental health challenges and undesirable behaviors. Mental illness can get in the way of your child behaving in a socially appropriate manner.

Following general parenting strategies may be helpful:

- Have a structured, predictable routine. Those of all ages who suffer from mental illnesses are vulnerable to disruptions and changes in their schedules. Aim for a schedule that is not too busy but not one with long periods of inactivity. On weekends and vacations, build in relaxing, soothing activities destined to relieve stress.

- Maintain a simple mood log or online journal. Identify mood patterns and triggers.

- Plan ahead or plan to fail. You cannot control everything, but whenever possible, avoid situations likely to trigger meltdowns. Prepare in advance. Let your child help.

- Troubleshoot to decrease family conflict. Pick your battles. Focus on deescalating conflicts and moods. Be calm and consistent. Set achievable limits and enforce them firmly. When it is realistic, involve your child in solving issues. Teach and model good problem-solving skills.

- Focus on the child's strengths. Encourage channeling energies into appropriate activities. Praise appropriate behaviors. Draw attention to the child's use of talents, skills, and positive traits.

- Know what is going on at school, at the park, and with friends. Talk with your child about these stressful situations. Brainstorm ways to manage them.

TAMU LEWIS

- Be aware of the difficulty of transitions. These include daily transitions, like going to bed, getting up, showering, and having breakfast, to major transitions, like starting school or going to a birthday party. Preplanning and rehearsals avoid embarrassing surprises.

- Monitor your teenager's friends and activities. Teens with bipolar issues are prime candidates for alcohol or drug abuse and other risky behaviors. Check use of cell phones, social media, and the internet.

- Always have a crisis plan. Practice fire drills, 911 call procedures, and crisis hotline numbers. Make sure there is a support person's number clearly posted where your child can see it. Make sure all the kids know the plans and procedures in place. It is especially important to have a well-thought-out and smoothly operating emergency plan because youngsters with bipolar issues are more likely than most to become violent or suicidal. The emergency plan should include plans for sibling safety.

- Avoid unrealistic expectations. Address your child's special needs. Set intermediate goals to work toward.

- As the parent of a child with bipolar disorder, your job is exhausting, stressful, and lonely. It is crucial to take time for yourself. Seek support from friends, family, or professional respite staff. See my chapter on self-care. Look into resources in the community, therapy, after school programs, and support groups.

Tips for Setting Realistic Expectations

As parents, you are your child's biggest supporters, coaches, and cheerleaders. You want your child to do well, so you set the bar high and encourage your child to leap over the hurdle.

In our exuberance, sometimes we set the bar too high. Setting the bar at just the right spot is an acquired skill. What should you consider?

Every child is unique. Before setting expectations, consider your child's interests, talents, and learning preferences.

Make sure the goals are age-appropriate. Check to see if this is something your child wants to do at all. Do some research to determine whether the activity is safe.

Remember, these are not *your* expectations. Don't set a high bar. If you excel at something, maybe your expectations for your child are too high. If you find something challenging, perhaps your expectations are too low.

Make sure your expectations are clear. Demonstrate. Create a list. Set milestones and celebrate each one.

Forget all-or-nothing. Work in steps. Encourage at every step.

POEM: BELIEVE IT AND SEE IT

Who would have thought
that moving out would lead to a 360 turnabout
of your thinking, being, and ways?

If I wasn't experiencing it for myself,
I wouldn't believe the days
that have followed the move.

You've grown up, and you're continuing to grow.
You do the things that I taught you
even though I thought you weren't taking the lessons in.

You tell me about what you're doing and what works for you.
It is all of the things I said.
You come visit often, and you actually enjoy spending time with
us, your family.

I'm like, whoa!
You used to prefer staying behind your closed bedroom door.

You still need support, but you talk it out
and manage not to get frazzled.
I'm amazed and thankful for that.

I know you will still experience ups and downs,
but that is life.

I pray that you stay on the path
that got you where you are today
and know that I am here,
rooting for you, always.

Useful Resources

Elaine Ho, "6 Parent Tips for Setting Goals with Your Child."
September 4, 2020, https://blog.edmentum.com

Joseph Klemz, "Parent Goal Setting Makes Better Parents."
December 6, 2021, https://reallifecounseling.us

Pamela Li, "3 Powerful Types of Parenting Goals That Will
Change Your Life." February 6, 2022, https://www.parent-
ingforbrain.com

Nicole Black, "8 Effective Parenting Goals to Make Your Life
Easier." December 1, 2021, https://messymotherhood.com

CHAPTER 7
Intentional Self-Care (Fifth Key)

Self-care is never a selfish act—it is simply good
stewardship of the only gift I have, the gift I was
put on earth to offer to others.
—Parker Palmer

SELF-CARE IS PROBABLY THE most important thing that
you can do to survive the mental health tank. When we think
about self-care, particularly as women, we may think of treating
ourselves. Maybe we think about the nail salon, a massage, a deli-
cious dessert, or going shopping at our favorite store.

According to Oxford Dictionary, self-care is "the practice of
taking an active role in protecting one's own well-being and hap-
piness, in particular during periods of stress."

I know we all agree. It's important to take care of ourselves.
But it's also incredibly hard to do so on a daily basis. We worry that
so many others around us need our care and attention. But here's

the thing: making time for ourselves isn't just nice—it's *necessary* for our well-being. We cannot be any good for others if we don't look after ourselves first!

I want to challenge you to go deeper and think about things that will actually serve you and nurture your inner self. Consider things that will restore you. And think about things that can be incorporated into your life on a regular basis and become routine practices.

Self-care will look different for different people. Think about what resonates with you. When I say, "Go deeper," I am referring to meditation. I know some people don't want to try meditation. They feel like they can't stop random thoughts from coming into their minds. In that case, you may want to try a guided meditation instead of just sitting in silence.

I do guided meditation every day. Contrary to what you may think, meditation doesn't have to be long to be beneficial. Sometimes, five or ten minutes can make a difference in terms of grounding you, putting you in touch with your inner self, and helping you get to a state of calm.

Importance of Breath Work

Another thing you might consider is breath work. Become aware of your breathing patterns. How does your breathing change if you are in a heightened state of stress? You may actually be holding your breath or breathing in a really shallow manner. Focus on taking some deep breaths. A simple practice is to pause and take six deep breaths. Try to breathe deeper each time that you breathe. Do that throughout your day or anytime you're feeling a heightened level of stress. This technique can be helpful when you're trying to figure something out or help your child or meet a work deadline.

There are many benefits to breath work awareness. These may include the following:

- Reduced stress

    - Breath work is a safe and effective way to cope with feelings like stress, anxiety, anger, grief, sadness, and depression. Long, deep breaths from the body's core calm, energize, ground, and focus the mind. Blood pressure and heart rate lower. Changing breathing changes brain waves. This decreases negative self-talk and increases optimistic thoughts.

- Increased energy

    - Breath work improves the amount of oxygen in the bloodstream. This increases energy, promotes stamina, and boosts your immune system.

- Improved self-awareness

    - Breathing through the mouth increases self-awareness. Focusing on the present brings higher levels of joy.

- Increased positive thoughts

    - Breath work allows us to shift away from negativity. The result is an increase in positive self-love.

- Improved sleep patterns

    - Breath work helps combat dietary and stress factors that impede sleep. You will fall asleep faster and get better sleep.

- Reduced trauma

    - Breath work helps process and eliminate bottled up negative emotions from your body. Breathing dislodges fears and paranoia, unravels dread, and blocks limiting self-talk.

- Eased pain

    - Chronic pain can be eased through conscious breathing. Breath work allows you to distance your body from pain and ignore it. This can even stimulate your body to heal itself.

- Released toxins

    - Deep breathing releases toxins. It also boosts lung efficiency. Over half of the toxins in your body can be expelled through effective breathing. They leave as part of carbon dioxide.

- Improved digestion

- Breathing stimulates blood flow in the digestive tract. It also reduces stress, which in turn reduces bloating and gas, improving digestive efficiency.

• Altered consciousness

- Through deep breathing, you can stimulate spiritual awareness and deepen your connection to yourself and others.

There are other helpful practices that you might consider to be more fun. These activities can also nurture your soul. Think about listening to music, dancing, or singing. You may like various forms of creativity like drawing, painting, performing, or playing an instrument.

If you're like me, you may have done some of these activities in your childhood. Then when you became an adult, you left these activities behind because of the business of life. I was a dancer when I was younger. I was a performer. I was always acting and singing in theater productions. Then in middle school and high school, I played the flute in the marching band. I performed in competitions. I performed solos and duets and won awards. Somehow, when I went off to college, I dropped it all.

Take a moment to think about it and get in touch with your inner child and what you may have left along the way that you enjoyed previously. Reflect on joyful activities from your childhood. Then make some time to incorporate some of those joyful activities into your present life.

When I say make some time, that's what I mean. Particularly as parents, and specifically moms, if you're like me, your schedule is hectic. You are always taking care of others. That is the nurturing aspect of mothers. You want things to get done, and you want things done right. A lot of the time, that leads to doing things yourself instead of delegating. However, let us not overlook the benefits of delegating.

I want you to put a spotlight on yourself. Focus on your self-care. Make an appointment with yourself. This is what I tell people all the time. Make an appointment with yourself—literally put it on your calendar—and do it.

I do things as simple as taking myself to the movies. When we were in a rough patch with my daughter's mental illness, I went to the movies by myself every other week. On a Tuesday night, I would let my husband know so he could come home and take care of the girls. I would prepare dinner in advance or ask my husband to cook. Going to the movies gave me a break. During the two hours when I was sitting in that movie theater by myself, I didn't have to worry about anyone else. I was completely engrossed in that movie. It was one of those theaters where they served food. So I could eat and watch that movie, and for two hours, all was well.

Figure out what works for you so that you can nurture yourself and allow yourself to reset. Once is not enough. It needs to be something that you enjoy that is simple to implement. Make sure it is not complicated and that it doesn't involve too many moving parts that may derail you. This allows you to commit to doing it on a regular basis. Whatever that is for you, figure it out and do it.

You know and I know that when you are stressed and tired, typically something else will go wrong in your body—at least that's the case with me. In the past, I would start having these illnesses or aches and pains or some condition would show up out of nowhere. When you're stressed, you typically don't sleep well. This compromises your immune system. Your immune system begins to break down and then you begin to feel even worse. So then what happens? If you're not feeling well, you're on edge. You have a low tolerance level. You are more easily agitated. You might find yourself snapping at your kids, your partner, and people at work, and that's not what you want to do. In that state, you are not showing up as your best self. I know as parents, as moms, as providers, as caregivers, as nurturers, that's the last thing you want to do. You do not want to go off on people for no reason—all because you didn't take care of yourself.

Reclaim yourself physically. It is easy to fall into a punishing pattern when you are overwhelmed by your situation. In a word, don't. Instead of reaching for the cookies, go for a long walk or join a gym. If you can afford to, hire a personal trainer to get you started on an exercise regimen.

Self-care fits into four categories: emotional, physical, psychological, and spiritual health. Let's look at examples of each:

- Physical self-care

  - This has to do with an overall healthy lifestyle. This includes things like eating healthily, drinking half of your body weight in ounces of water a day (e.g., if you weigh 150 pounds, you should drink 75 ounces of water daily), and getting at least thirty minutes of exercise every day.

- Emotional self-care

  - This might include setting clear, unwavering boundaries on your time. It also involves preserving your energy and learning to say no without guilt. Surround yourself with positive people. Give yourself affirmative and inspiring messages. Deal with issues or problems immediately so that they don't build up. Send out and receive messages of love, kindness, and support. Spend time with caring, genuinely kind people.

- Psychological self-care

  - Psychological self-care activities might include personal and professional education and development. Give attention to personal reflection. Note your inner experiences. Examine your inner thoughts and feelings. Engage in activities that build self-awareness, such as journaling, keeping a feelings diary, seeking feedback from others, engaging in meditation, or seeking out coaching or counseling. Look for activities that give you a chance to grow as a person, to learn new skills or new information, and to reflect.

- Spiritual self-care

  - This might include prayer or meditation. Try guided visualization. Practice gratitude. Go for walks. Spend time in nature. Become aware of the nonmaterial aspects of your life. Decide what is meaningful to you. Be in the moment. Practice mindfulness.

Even though you may feel like you have everything that you need, you need to build in self-care—if not for you, then for others around you.

Think about this: What is it that you need to improve?

We may have some challenging things on our plate, and they have to get done, and we have to be the one to do all these things. That's the story that we tell ourselves. And to be honest, that is our comfort zone—just to be doing, going, serving.

You need to be honest with yourself by going within, looking at yourself, and determining your workload.

It may not sound all that appealing. Somehow, you may think that if you actually need this self-care, it somehow makes you less than competent. This is, of course, completely false. That's some story that you made up that you tell yourself. You imagine people are going to think that you can't handle everything.

Face it! People are not even worried about you because they have their own problems, okay? They're not thinking about you. All they know is what they see—you are always doing something. So if you said no, N-O, every once in a while, they might be surprised, but they would be able to find another person or resource to fulfill their request.

Saying no is not going to change someone's perception of you. That's just the story that you tell yourself to stay in that comfort zone where you burn yourself out. I'm here to tell you that at some point, your body will say, "Hell to the no" on your behalf.

Your body will break down on you. I know what I'm talking about. I know from experience. That is not what you want. My body is quick to tell me. Sometimes, in the past, I have ignored it. I have ignored it and then ended up in a bad situation with operations and surgeries and recoveries.

If I'm sitting in the hospital, then I certainly can't help my child or my family, right? It's like a vicious cycle. We tell ourselves, "Hey! I don't have time to nurture myself and take care of myself because I'm doing this stuff for all these other people."

But if you end up sick in bed, you can't do anything for anybody. You have basically just shot yourself in the foot, as they say. You haven't done any good for anybody, and now you—along with everybody else—must figure out what to do next since you are now sick in bed. We want to avoid that. Look at it this way: if you model positive self-care for your children and your family members—so they see you taking care of yourself, taking a break, meditating, exercising—then that makes it okay for them to do that too. You would be not only creating these healthy habits for yourself but also creating them for the next generation, for your children and their children. How powerful is that?

And we all know that even though our children may treat us like we're old and we don't know anything, they are watching everything we do, and they hear everything that we say, whether or not they actually agree with it. In real time, they are hearing it. They are sponges, and they are seeing it. If you want to set a good example for them, you need to be a role model in terms of self-care, and then they can avoid the burnout that is so prevalent among moms and, really, all women in our society.

I know it is hard for some of you to put yourself first. If you don't want to do it for yourself, do it for your children and their children. Take care of yourself so you can show up as your best self for yourself and for your family. You might find that somewhere down the road, sooner or later, practicing and modeling positive self-care allows you to experience more peace and harmony in your life. Instead of serving your family from a state of frustration and exhaustion, you will be refreshed and restored with the fuel to do what you want to do.

There may be things you want to accomplish for yourself: a business you want to start, a desired promotion at work, or a hobby you want to pick up. There might be a place where you want to volunteer and serve others. There may be someone you want to mentor. What you'll find is once you begin to take better care of yourself, typically it becomes easier to help those around you because now you've built yourself up. Now you actually have something to give from your overflow. Release the pressure that you feel from the pressure cooker that you've put yourself in. When you take care of yourself, that strain and pressure is relieved. You have a new perspective, and typically people just inherently, by osmosis, recognize that you're coming from a different place. Because you are acting differently, they respond differently. You're coming from a place of an abundance of self-care, and being able to serve from that overflow looks different. It comes out differently. It doesn't come off as an obligation or something that's necessary for you to do. All these things benefit everybody—not just you. This allows you to come from a happy place. You may experience multiple benefits from taking care of yourself.

Is there one perfect self-care activity? Any activity that makes you feel more relaxed, helps to reduce symptoms of stress and anxiety, and lifts your mood is an ideal self-care activity for you right now. Why not get daring and try something new?

One of the ways to build time for self-care is to delegate. You can't do everything yourself. Even if you'd do it better, self-care requires that you loosen the controls and let others do things.

Benefits of Delegating

- Delegation plays an important role in self-care.

- Delegation is more efficient. By transferring tasks to others, you buy yourself time for activities like self-care. It also lessens your stress and fatigue.

- Delegation develops others' talents, confidence, and responsibility. This improves their relationship with you.

- By delegating, you are nurturing and coaching. Others build new skills and feel better about themselves as you delegate responsibilities to them. As a mentor or coach, you learn new skills and foster a greater self-concept.

- Delegation gives you the time to focus on other tasks.

- Delegation increases trust and communication among you and those to whom you delegate.

- Delegation improves productivity and time management.

Self-Care Activities

Not all self-care activities fit into the "pampering" category. In fact, there are multiple aspects of self-care:

- Physical
- Psychological
- Emotional
- Social
- Professional
- Environmental
- Spiritual
- Financial

The American Psychological Association defines self-care as "those activities that contribute to physical, mental, and psychological wellness." The National Institute of Health says that self-care is an individual's attempts to promote good health, detect symptoms of poor health at an early stage, prevent illness, and manage chronic conditions.

Given these parameters, physical self-care activities may include a long-term physical regimen of getting exercise, eating a nutritious diet, attending regular checkups, taking baths or showers, drinking lots of water, getting eight hours of uninterrupted sleep, sitting in the sun, or going for a walk.

Psychological self-care activities may include creative arts, meditation, deep breathing, reading a book, guided visualization, or listening to music.

When you consciously practice emotional self-care, you might delegate duties, say no to requests, take time for reflecting, and become aware of your emotional boundaries.

Social self-care involves having a supportive group and social network. Social self-care might include engaging in regular social activities with friends, seeking help for a project, spending time with family or friends, and getting out to meet new people through church groups or clubs.

Professional self-care involves sharing skills or strengths with others in mentorships or attending professional development opportunities like conferences or meetings or listening to podcasts.

The importance of environmental self-care is often overlooked. It includes neat, organized, and well-maintained home and work environments. Examples of environmental self-care include decluttering, time management, good hygiene, and a clean, safe living environment.

Spiritual self-care is not always about organized religion. It is all about the beliefs and values that guide your life. Spiritual self-care may include keeping a gratitude diary, going on a retreat, bird-watching, meditating, or enjoying a sunset.

Financial self-care involves making conscious money management decisions. Financial self-care activities include knowing your financial status, budgeting responsibly, paying bills on time, spending judiciously, and investing wisely.

What Research Says about Self-Care

Research has indicated that self-care eases stress and improves your physical, mental, and emotional well-being. Through increased self-care, individuals increase their resilience. Those who consistently practice self-care also increase their life span and positive outlook on life.

Get Connected

I encourage you to get started with your self-care routine right now. Check in with me at https://www.facebook.com/groups/parenting-supporttribe, and let me know how it is going. You can download my free mental wellness guide at https://tamulewis.com/freegift/. You can also connect with me at https://www.ltyfoundation.org to stay updated on our latest mental health education initiatives. I encourage you to be intentional about taking care of your physical and your mental health.

Useful Resources

Lesley Berk, "Development of Guidelines for Caregivers of People with Bipolar Disorder: A Delphi expert consensus study." December 1, 2021, https://pubmed.ncbi.nlm.nih.gov

Lee Boag, "The Development and Evaluation of a Self-Care Intervention for Informal Caregivers of Relatives with Bipolar Disorder." August 15, 2016, http://hdl.handle. net/10059/1566

Brene` Brown, *I Thought it was Just Me*, (Garden City: Avery, 2007)

Julie Fast, *Loving Someone with Bipolar Disorder*, (New York: New Harbinger Publications, 2012)

Deborah Perlick, et al. "Randomized Trial Comparing Caregiver-Only Family-Focused Treatment to Standard Health Education on the 6-month Outcome of Bipolar Disorder." March 1, 2018, http://dx.doi.org/10.1111/ bdi.12621

Mike Robbins, *Nothing Changes until You Do*, (Carlsbad: Hay House Inc., 2015)

CHAPTER 8
Education Is Key

Having a mental disorder isn't easy, and it's even
harder when people assume you can just
get over it.
—HeathyPlace.com

YOU MIGHT HAVE FRIENDS who look at your child with a
mental illness with frustration, muttering or thinking, "Just get
over it!"

Having a mental illness is like being born with blue eyes or
having a stutter. People do not realize that having bipolar disorder
is not something you can "get over" or "outgrow" or "work around."

So how can you combat the deliberate or unintentional os-
tracism and the stigma surrounding those who live with mental
illnesses?

There is always a stigma surrounding "differences," including
physical and mental traits, outside any group's "normal" range of
thinking. Sometimes this comes from a lack of understanding.

There may even be irrational fears about the condition being contagious.

As I mentioned earlier, stigma most often comes from a lack of understanding. As humans, we frequently fear anything we don't understand.

When it comes to mental illnesses like bipolar disorder, the stigma is even stronger. People fear physical confrontation. Both the low and high periods are frightening to outsiders. Because of medications used to control the highs and lows, some parents fear a drug connection.

What are the Solutions?

As with anything at the school, in the neighborhood or your town or city, residents don't understand. Education—both formal and informal—is the key.

Learning everything you can about mental illness from a variety of sources is the first step.

Armed with reliable information, your next step is to help others understand. This may seem like an impossible task. It's like the saying goes, when eating an elephant, take one bite at a time.

Good things will come from your efforts. Your child will gain valuable strategies for coping with the illness. They will be more accepted in the family, the school, the neighborhood, and the community when more people know and are more comfortable with this condition.

Is this a scary venture? Of course it is! But you will do it for your child and for your family. Knowledge is the first step on the road to understanding and eventual acceptance.

As you begin your crusade, remember to take baby steps. Humans need several repetitions before they "get" things. Look for ways to present your message in a variety of ways.

You will learn some new technical skills, and you will be providing education for your family, your friends, your child's school, your neighborhood, and the community. It will be empowering for everyone—including you!

How Can You Help Educate Others?

First, get your facts and resources together. Be prepared to answer questions and direct people to helpful resources. If you are interested in presenting helpful information yourself, you can prepare an engaging presentation. Make good use of PowerPoint slides and photos. Be sure to tell your audience why you are doing this and what you hope to accomplish. People love human interest stories. Practice in front of the mirror. Branch out to family and friends. When you feel comfortable, look for audiences. Never lose sight of your goal. Like Johnny Appleseed, share your message one group at a time.

Accept offers to speak. I've been to early morning breakfasts to share mental health education with parents. I've been asked to speak at luncheons, community weekend themed days, and evening information nights at local schools. I accept them all. I speak within their time frame and build my network with new contacts at every opportunity. My family is supportive of my speaking engagements. I am enjoying the journey, helping others, and meeting some very interesting people along the way.

Don't just sit around like that wallflower. See an opportunity and invite yourself. Register as a speaker at local community groups, libraries, schools, churches, and service clubs.

Make social media your friend. If you do not have a presence on Facebook, Instagram, Twitter, and other useful platforms, get one. Start small. Dream big. Get yourself technical support from someone who champions your cause.

Sure! There are biases and stigmas surrounding mental illness or living with someone who has been diagnosed with a mental illness. But you can be the change you want to see! You can start with your family and extended family. This will make a difference to the people who interact with your child the most. It is perfectly fine if you prefer not to take on the task of educating the public. You can make a positive impact in your own circles by sharing your experiences and helpful information through natural conversations. If you are interested in taking your mental health advocacy further, you can take on the challenge to educate the public, your child's educators, and your neighbors. Just do whatever resonates with you, one step at a time.

Bipolar Misinformation

People with this disorder can have significant mood shifts where they feel and behave very differently. However, the symptoms of bipolar disorder can vary widely, and this leads to misinformation.
—Isabelle Morley

It is little wonder that those who do not live with bipolar disorder are confused. When I started to do my research for blogs and presentations, I was amazed and shocked at what I discovered.

Because bipolar disorder comes with an aura of mystery, it has a higher-than-usual set of these myths, half-truths, and misunderstandings. Here are a few myths and half-truths I discovered.

Bipolar Disorder Is Not a Real Disease

Is bipolar disorder just a more acceptable way of explaining extremes in behavior?

Formerly called manic-depressive illness, bipolar disorder is recognized by mental health associations around the world. Bipolar disorder is a mental disorder. It causes extreme shifts in mood, energy, activity, concentration, and productivity. In severe cases, those with bipolar disorder are unable to carry out daily tasks at home or at work.

You Can Get Tested for Bipolar Disorder

That's a myth of the first order. There is no test for bipolar disorder. Doctors consider such things as symptoms and medical history. There may be tests to eliminate other conditions with similar symptoms.

Sometimes bipolar diagnosis is a matter of "well, it isn't this or that other mental disorder, so it must be bipolar disorder."

Highs and Lows Can Be Controlled

This is a half-truth. While the extremes can often be mitigated with carefully monitoring, complete control is an often unattainable goal. That does not mean you ever give up on achieving that goal.

Highs and Lows Occur in Predictable Patterns

For most, bipolar disorder isn't nearly that tidy. In fact, for some people, symptoms of both mania and depression can occur at the same time.

Some people have one episode and don't have another for months or years. For others, highs and lows can occur one after the other in the space of a day. Usually, symptoms don't happen in a regular pattern.

If You're Experiencing Highs and Lows, It's Because You Aren't Taking Your Medication

Well, that may be the case, but in a lot of situations, the medication may need to be changed or tweaked. Symptoms change. People's bodies change.

Bipolar Is Bipolar—You Either Have It or You Don't

There is more than one type of bipolar. Symptoms, patterns, and even severity all differ.

There are a few different types of the disease. These can be categorized according to symptoms. Bipolar I is characterized by manic episodes or depressive episodes of over two weeks. Bipolar II episodes aren't as severe. In the cases of cyclothymic bipolar disorder, the highs and lows are mild. Unspecified bipolar disorder is the category used when the symptoms do not fit the other three categories, but episodes of unusual manic behavior are still present.

There's Only One Way to Treat Bipolar Disorder

Different treatment plans work for different people. For some people, medications work well to moderate highs and lows. The age of onset, the severity of the bipolar disorder, and the patient reaction to specific drugs are factors that must be considered when considering treatment options. Some people find great benefit from participating in individual therapy, group therapy, family therapy, and/or support groups.

Treating Bipolar Leads to Continued Drug Use

Patients diagnosed with bipolar are often on medication to stabilize their mood. They may also be prescribed antimanic drugs, antidepressants, and sleep enhancement drugs. There is no evidence to suggest that those with bipolar are more likely to take illegal drugs.

Kids Never Get Bipolar

There are documented bipolar disorder cases in children as young as six. Other children and teens may have been misdiagnosed as having ADHD. The two share symptoms and are equally difficult to diagnose.

Generally, diagnoses occur in the late teens and the early to midtwenties. Some cases don't appear until much later in life, around the age of fifty.

Genetics Have No Role in Bipolar Disorder

Your genetics may predispose you to bipolar disorder. However, many with bipolar have no family history of it.

A Bipolar Disorder Protects You from Other Mental Illnesses

A comforting thought, but many people with bipolar disorder have other mental health issues, including anxiety, anorexia, ADHD, or substance abuse.

Stress Isn't a Factor

Stressful events can act as triggers for bipolar symptoms, depression periods, or manic episodes.

Bipolar Disorder Diagnoses Are Rare
Almost 3 percent of American adults had bipolar disorder symptoms in 2020. Diagnoses have increased significantly—especially in children and teens.

The Cause of Bipolar Is Evident
In spite of significant research, a single cause of bipolar has not yet been found. Certain factors like stress, genetic makeup, and brain chemicals are being studied as possible causes.

People with Bipolar Disorder Are Just Moody
The extreme highs and lows that those with bipolar disorder experience could never be described as mere moodiness.

Bipolar Disorder Is Mostly Giddiness
Mania is a part of bipolar disorder, but its length and severity should not be considered giddiness.

The Manic Phase of Bipolar Is Enjoyable
For both the person with bipolar disorder and their associates, the manic period is full of energy and perhaps risky behavior. Mania can also manifest as irritability, edginess, sarcasm, feelings of lack of control, and restlessness.

There Is No Need for Medication after Bipolar Disorder Is under Control
Sadly, too many people feel this way! Bipolar medication is used to prevent the highs and the lows. Medication should never be stopped or altered without consulting a doctor.

How Myths Hurt Those Who Suffer from Bipolar

Because bipolar disorder has so many half-truths surrounding it, those who do not have direct contact frequently misunderstand it.

Misinformation feeds stigma and bias. The best way to deal with this is to use every opportunity to educate community members about bipolar disorder.

What's the harm in myths and misinformation? To answer this, let's take a look at what happened with COVID-19. Misinformation was so prevalent that while people were dying around them, there were still those who insisted COVID-19 was a hoax. As early as 2020, over 30 percent of Americans believed COVID-19 was a bioweapon created by China. A quarter of North Americans believed COVID-19 was intentionally planned.

Research shows that behaviors and attitudes surround belief in the need or non need for protective measures like mask wearing.

Some regarded measures to get the virus under control as fake news.

"The fundamental problem with misinformation is that once people have heard it, they tend to believe and act on it, even after it's been corrected," stated Dr. Stephan Lewandowsky, a professor of psychology at the University of Bristol.

Misinformation is not an easy task to fight. Sometimes, the harder you fight it, the stronger it seems to dig in.

Like with COVID-19, even after misinformation about bipolar disorder is corrected, false beliefs can still persist.

New information, even with indisputable proof, is often viewed as a ploy. Our thoughts can maintain a bias—even when we accept the new information as factual.

So, faced with solid evidence that bipolar disorder is not a mood or a personality flaw but rather a real mental illness, many still believe people can "get over it" or "snap out of it" or "rise above it" if they just put their mind to it.

Faced with these perceptions, it is hard for those who are trying to manage bipolar disorder to feel good about themselves. They get no credit for the gains they are making in their fight against bipolar disorder.

It's the same battle fought by those with drug, alcohol, and gambling addictions. These, too, are seen as personal flaws, not illnesses. People who suffer from these illnesses are often seen as morally or physically weak.

It takes a long time and a lot of repetition to correct misinformation. It's like a bad habit. Breaking it is much harder than developing the right habit in the first place. The answer is not to throw up our hands and give up. It's to take the advice of people like Martin Luther King Jr. and Gandhi and continue to fight.

POEM: I'M STILL SAD

It's been five years, and I'm still sad.
I guess you could say I'm still mad
on some level, on some days,
because I feel like he tried
to let others know what he was feeling inside,
but the mental illness took him and moved him aside.

We didn't get it,
Not really,
even though we were by his side,
not until after the fact,
so we weren't able to prevent the act,
so he died by suicide.
What?
Yes, suicide.

Now others are still suffering,
still battling, still fighting, still trying to climb that mountain
each day,
and I just wish someone would find a way
to make it easier for them and their loved ones every day.

All I can do is continue to give my best, and
I pray
for an everlasting solution
to this thing called mental illness and all of its confusion.

Useful Resource

Anthony Wilkenson, *Bipolar Disorder: Understanding Symptoms, Mood Swings, and Treatment,* (Unknown: Independent Publishing, 2014)

CHAPTER 9
Setting Up a Lifetime Management and Treatment Plan

> Recovery is not one and done. It is a lifelong
> journey that takes place one day,
> one step at a time.
> —Unknown

What Is a Lifetime Management and Treatment Plan?

THOSE WHO HAVE BEEN diagnosed with bipolar disorder have ongoing needs. From the outset, their symptoms are going to have to be assessed. The medical team and psychiatric team will meet with the patient. Their conversation will center around the best medication to regulate manic and depressive periods and the best therapy to address mental health issues.

These health-care professionals are tasked with making the life of the individual as smooth, supported, and productive as possible.

There is a good reason why those with bipolar disorder need a treatment team. Bipolar disorder, once diagnosed, is a lifelong condition. Hence, those who have it need a lifetime management and treatment team. This group of medical professionals will offer integrated, multidisciplinary services to meet the unpredictable challenges that bipolar disorder presents. The disorder often runs an unpredictable course of ups and downs.

The presence of the team is critical. If bipolar disorder is left untreated, those highs and lows will be left unregulated. The results could be—and often are—devastating. Recurring manic and depressive episodes that characterize bipolar disorder, if not medicated, make it difficult to lead a stable life. Having a productive livelihood may be a distant dream without the monitoring and intervention of the lifetime management and treatment team.

In the manic phase, a person may be hyperactive and irresponsible. In the depressive phase, it may be difficult to do anything at all.

Early diagnosis and treatment are key. Moreover, the successful treatment of bipolar disorder depends on several factors.

Medication can be vital, but as any of us who have tried to navigate medication know, it can be a tricky path. Medication alone is not nearly enough.

Treatment also involves knowing about yourself or your family member who suffer from bipolar disorder.

No matter how much you monitor signs and educate yourself about medication and alternative approaches, you still need to communicate with your doctors and therapists.

Don't try to do this alone! You need the advice and expertise of a strong support system.

It is also vital that the person with bipolar disorder and their caregivers help themselves by making healthy lifestyle choices. They need to be in the best physical and emotional health possible to navigate this journey. Being in the best shape may also help reduce the person's need for medication.

Treatment plans should be created by the management team, including the client and their caregivers. Once it is in place, it is important to stick to the treatment plan. If it needs to be reassessed, that happens with the management team. Sure! Changes will need to happen as changes in life and the body occur. The point I'm trying to make here is this: think of the body as a finely tuned machine, and think of any medication or alternative approaches as the fuel that machine runs on. You're not the expert on either of these, so don't mess with them. Give the information to the management team and trust in their expertise to make needed changes to the treatment plan.

Effectively managing mental illness doesn't happen overnight. There is no finite cure or management plan. In fact, recovery isn't in the cards. Don't delude yourself. Just as the mood swings of bipolar disorder have their ups and downs, so, too, does the treatment plan have ups and downs.

It takes time to find the right treatment plan. Acknowledge the fact that setbacks will happen.

With careful supervision by the life management team and with trust and commitment from the person and their caregivers, you, like our daughter Nya, can get your symptoms under control. The goal of the life management team is that the person lives life to the fullest.

What Is Family Therapy?

As I have mentioned on several occasions throughout this book, I am a big proponent of family therapy. It has saved our family on numerous occasions.

Family therapy, also called family counseling, is a type of psychotherapy. Its goal is to identify family patterns that contribute to a behavior disorder or mental illness like bipolar. Family therapists then help family members break those habits or replace them with better ones. Family therapists use discussion and problem-solving in working with families.

Types of Family Therapy

- Structural therapy

  - The theory was developed by Salvador Minuchin. Structural therapy focuses on interactions between people. It is based on family dynamics. A family therapist aims to help the family outgrow constraining growth patterns and develop as a new and stronger entity.

- Strategic therapy

  - Strategic therapy has evolved from a number of psychotherapy practices. The parts include the social stage, the problem stage, the interactional stage, the goal-setting stage, and the task-setting stage.

- Systemic therapy

  - This therapy is rooted in looking at the family as a system. Systemic therapy approaches problems in a social reality.

- Narrative therapy

  - Narrative therapy encourages everyone's individuality. They are then challenged to employ their skill set to deal with family problems and minimize them.

  - In life, people create personal stories. These help them to decide who they are and what tools they possess to navigate their lives. Narrative therapy helps clarify, develop, support, and guide people on life's journey.

- Transgenerational therapy

  - Therapists have the ability to observe interactions between individuals across multiple generations. Their observations and analyses help get at the core issues of the family group. Concepts of transgenerational therapy help create a lens through which to frame the issue being addressed.

- Communication therapy

  - The failure to communicate is a common problem in most families. There may be differences in cultural backgrounds or personal experiences. Issues like bipolar disorder add another layer of stress and trauma and heighten communication issues. A trained therapist can help families decide on the best strategies for improving communication. Skills might include honest dialogue, active listening, opening lines of communication, and mediated communication.

- Psychoeducation

    - This involves helping families with mental health conditions empower and support themselves. This is a strong tool against bias, stigmatization, and prejudice surrounding mental health conditions.

- Relationship counseling

    - Relationships are hard. Daily problems strain relationships. Add bipolar disorder, and the highs and lows of this mental illness can cause irreconcilable differences.

    - Often called "couple's counseling," relationship counseling isn't just for couples. It is a type of talk therapy where the parties in a relationship talk about their problems and feelings. Either in person or online, a trained therapist offers a safe and private venue.

    - Participants in relationship therapy have a chance to talk through their problems. The result is a better understanding of themselves. They can often make changes that improve their relationships.

- Trained counselors listen actively and help people deal with negative thoughts and feelings. They use techniques like conflict resolution, behavior counseling, life coaching, positive self-talk, and hypnotherapy.

- In seeking the best therapist for your needs, ask how they would treat a specific issue. Ask them about their typical procedures and mediation session steps.

What Is Family Focused Therapy?

The therapist works to educate family members about mental illness issues and how these impact them both individually and as a family unit.

Family therapy techniques are focused on giving families improved communication skills, minimizing stress, increasing problem-solving strategies, and helping families work together in harmony.

Family focused therapy sessions teach participants to do the following:

• Identify symptoms and triggers
• Employ more effective communication skills
• Resolve conflicts
• Use problem-solving skills
• Learn constructive solutions to mental illness issues

Is Family Therapy Effective?

Those involved in family therapy usually avoid relapses and hasten recovery from bipolar episodes.

Depressive symptoms are eased by family therapy.

Useful Resources

Alan Carr, "The Evidence Base for Family Therapy and Systemic Interventions for Child-Focused Problems," *Journal of Family Therapy.* Issue 36, Volume 2 (2014) 107–157.

Matthew McKay, *Mind and Emotions,* (Oakland: New Harbinger, 2011)

David Miklowitz and Bowen Chung, "Family-Focused Therapy for Bipolar Disorder: Reflections on 30 Years of Research." July 29, 2016, https://pubmed.ncbi.nlm.nih.gov/27471058/

Sheri Van Dijk, *Calming the Emotional Storm,* (Oakland: New Harbinger Publications, 2012)

Advocacy

I learned a long time ago the wisest thing I can do is be on my own side, be an advocate for myself and others like me.

—Maya Angelou

What Is Advocacy?

In advocacy, individuals or groups support and influence political, economic, and social decisions. The goal of an advocate is to gain support in a certain environment to create change for the better.

Why Is Advocacy Important?

Like in *The Lorax*, advocates speak for those who cannot speak for themselves.

A culture and creativity study notes that if only 10 percent of a population holds a strong belief, they can persuade the rest to adopt a belief.

With the right amount of support, help, and a common goal, you can change the way the world views bipolar disorder and those who live with it.

If we advocate strongly, people around the world will have better health care, live freely, and be treated equally.

Advocacy is not new. Advocates have been contributing to the world's success for centuries. Advocates come from different backgrounds and places, but they share a common goal. They want to improve specific situations.

Ways to Advocate for Those Living with Bipolar Disorder

- Become a volunteer in an organization that actively helps those with bipolar disorder or their families. These might include:

  - Depression and Bipolar Support Alliance: https://www.dbsalliance.org/

  - Substance Abuse and Mental Health Services Administration: https://www.samhsa.gov/find-help/national-helpline

  - National Alliance on Mental Illness: https://www.nami.org

  - Mental Health America: https://www.healthline.com/health/mental-health/bipolar-support-groups#mha

  - Daily Strength: https://www.healthline.com/health/mental-health/bipolar-support-groups#dailystrength

- Make a donation or organize fundraising activities for groups that support individuals with mental illness and their families.

  - Good examples include the Sean Costello Memorial Fund for Bipolar Research, Music Benefit Concerts, and sponsoring therapy sessions for those in need.

- Donations can support research regarding the methods to identify and treat mental illness.

- Educate yourself and others about bipolar disorder through seminars, conferences, courses, podcasts, videos, books, articles, and programs.

- Read about and discover resources for managing bipolar disorder. Consider becoming part of research studies or clinical trials.

- Help a friend or a family living with bipolar disorder.

- Approach a business, organization, or enterprise to sponsor infomercials about bipolar disorder and beneficial techniques.

- Start a blog or post helpful information about bipolar disorder on other people's sites.

How Can You Help Your Child Self-Advocate?

While it is important to advocate, it is more important to teach your child how to advocate for themself. Try these strategies:

- Reassure your child that they will be heard by their audience, whether that be an educator, health-care provider, classmate, neighbor, family member, or friend. Then pave the way for this to happen. Gradually allow your child to take the lead in self-advocacy.

- Encourage your child to reach out to others and ask for help.

- Encourage your child to listen to their body, mind, and emotions and to give themselves what they need.

- Nurture self-confidence and self-acceptance.

- Encourage your child to do their homework before beginning self-advocacy projects.

POEM: I CHOOSE *YOU*

Even when I'm frustrated, angry, hurt, and upset,
I love you unconditionally.
You can place that bet.

This journey with you has taught me many lessons…exercise,
flex my skills,
patience,
humility,
compromise,
listening,
quiet,
trusting,
letting go.
I have to go to therapy too
just to make it through
to help myself and you,
but you know what?
I don't mind.
I do what I need to do
because I choose *you.*

You ask us not to care.
You ask us not to be there,
but I know that's not really the truth.

Please, Nya, choose *you.*

Useful Resources

Steven Hayes, *Get Out of Your Mind and Into Your Life: The New Acceptance and Commitment Therapy*, (Oakland: New Harbinger, 2005)

Kevin Connolly, "The Clinical Management of Bipolar Disorder: A Review of Evidence-Based Guidelines." May 5, 2010, https://pubmed.ncbi.nlm.nih.gov/22132354/

Michael Jann, "Diagnosis and Treatment of Bipolar Disorders in Adults: A Review of the Evidence on Pharmacologic Treatments." December 1, 2014, https://www.ncbi.nlm.nih.gov/pmc/articles/PMC4296286/

Michael Otto, *Managing Bipolar*, (Oxford: Oxford University Press, 2008)

Conclusion

Your illness is not your identity. Your chemistry
is not your character.
—Rick Warren

NEARLY 3 PERCENT OF the population has been diagnosed with bipolar disorder. Of these, almost 85 percent of them fall in the severe range. We can only speculate about how many more have not been identified or were misdiagnosed.

This book is not a pity party. I have shared my personal story to help those with bipolar disorder cope with their symptoms and reach out for help. I believe that if we all better understand mental illness, we can support one another.

How can you help? You've taken a very important first step. By reading my book, you've shown you care. You've indicated a readiness to help those thousands who suffer—often alone—with bipolar disorder.

Programs and initiatives that educate the public help us understand signs and treatments for bipolar disorder. A clearer, wider understanding builds empathy and dispels the stigma around this little-known illness.

MENTAL HEALTH RESOURCES

- American Foundation for Suicide Prevention
  - www.suicidepreventionlifeline.org
  - 800-273-TALK (8255)

- Depression and Bipolar Support Alliance (DBSA)
  - www.dbsalliance.org
  - 800-826-3632

- The Jed Foundation
  - www.jedfoundation.org
  - 212-647-7544

- Mental Health America (MHA)
  - www.nmha.org
  - 800-969-6642

- National Alliance on Mental Illness (NAMI)
  - www.nami.org
  - 800-950-NAMI (6264)

- Lee Thompson Young Foundation
  - www.ltyfoundation.org
  - 678-444-4566

- Sunovion Answers
  - 855-5LATUDA

Unfortunately, the media continues to portray individuals with bipolar disorder as insane, out of control, dangerous, or criminal. This misinformation contributes to problems with bipolar disorder behaviors and acquiring necessary treatment. We need to campaign for media depictions that are accurate so that coping with the condition will encourage treatment.

Those who are dealing with bipolar disorder need a range of treatments that may include medication, support groups, and psychotherapy. They need help dealing with negative feelings. They need reassurance that their mental illness doesn't define them.

People aren't mentally ill. They have a mental illness diagnosis. This distinction can make a world of difference to an individual coping with a condition and how they view themselves.

There is a need for more mental health research, policy changes, and advocacy groups. These are essential to improving both the lives and the treatment outcomes for those coping with bipolar disorder.

If fear can become understanding and compassion one person at a time, we can improve life for those with bipolar disorder.

We're all different. Rather than focusing on these differences, if we celebrate the strengths and uniqueness of each human being and treat others without judgment, we can make the world a better place. Listen to the struggles of those around you. Reach out a helping hand. Let others know you've been there and you understand. That was more helpful to me on my journey than anything else.

Modern technology has created a lifeline for those living with bipolar disorder. Thanks to Zoom and other virtual platforms, we can interact with the life management team almost immediately. It is so comforting for both Nya and our family to know these professionals have our backs when things take a downward turn.

My social media followers have given me hope and good ideas. I am so grateful to them and to the technology that connects us.

What does the future hold for those diagnosed as bipolar? First, more work needs to be done on the diagnosis process. It takes too long, and the disorder is frequently misdiagnosed because it shares symptoms with other illnesses like ADHD. A psychiatrist may compare symptoms with the documented criteria for bipolar and related disorders in the Diagnostic and Statistical Manual of Mental Disorders (DSM-5), published by the American Psychiatric Association. Some mental health professionals use psychological assessments and questionnaires, which may occur over a period of several days or weeks. Time is of the essence to try to regulate the highs and lows of bipolar disorder. Inroads are being made using biomarkers to speed up identification and suggest a personal treatment plan.

As for treatment? The availability of multiple treatments and carefully constructed treatment plans give those living with bipolar disorder hope that—while not being cured—they can get better and stay better. Thanks to the efforts of life management teams, those who deal with bipolar disorder can now function well between episodes and control the extremes of the highs and lows during episodes.

We've come a long way. Today, between 70 and 80 percent of people with bipolar disorder are receiving treatment that controls mood swings enough for them to work and have meaningful relationships. Another 20 to 30 percent still struggle to maintain a fulfilling life.

There is no cure for bipolar disorder, but increasing numbers have been able to manage their symptoms and lead productive lives.

> Mental health problems don't define who you are.
> They are something you experience. You walk in
> the rain and you feel the rain, but, importantly,
> YOU ARE NOT THE RAIN.
> —Matt Haig

Glossary of Terms

Acute: Short but severe.

Adjunctive: In addition to the main treatment.

Affective disorder: Depression, bipolar disorder, and seasonal affective disorder.

Akathisia: A state of agitation, distress, and severe restlessness that may be an occasional side-effect of medication.

Anticonvulsant: Medications developed primarily to prevent epileptic seizures.

Antidepressant: A class of medications effective in treating the symptoms of depression.

Antipsychotic: A class of medications originally developed to reduce the frequency and the severity of psychotic episodes. The newer atypical or second-generation antipsychotics are used to treat bipolar disorder or more severe depression. Many people who take these medications don't have psychotic symptoms.

Bipolar disorder (also known as manic depression): A psychiatric condition characterized by extreme mood states of mania and depression. A person may have bipolar disorder even if they have experienced only one of the extreme mood states, making diagnosis very challenging.

Bipolar I: A type of bipolar disorder characterized by at least one full-blown manic episode not medically attributable to medication or substance abuse.

Bipolar II: Bipolar disorder characterized by one or more major depressive episodes not medically attributable to another cause. One or more hypomanic episodes occurs. Chronic depression is usually more problematic than the hypomania. Full manic episodes change the diagnosis to bipolar I.

Bipolar not otherwise specified (NOS): Also known as unspecified bipolar and related disorder. A type of bipolar disorder characterized by hypomanic, manic, or depressive episodes that don't fit in any of the other bipolar categories and can't be ascribed to unipolar depression.

Catatonia: A state of profound lack of movement and language, often including odd or unusual physical and verbal responses to stimuli. Sometimes alternates with periods of agitation and overexcitement. Can be associated with bipolar disorder, unipolar depression, schizophrenia, and other psychiatric and medical conditions.

Circadian rhythm: Biological pattern of sleep, wakefulness, and energy that plays out through the course of a day. Some studies show that irregularities in a person's circadian rhythm can destabilize moods.

Cognitive behavioral therapy (CBT): Therapy that works at the intersection between thoughts, feelings, and behavior. The therapist teaches concepts and strategies to the client, who practices new skills between sessions. Studies show that CBT is effective for treating depression, anxiety, obsessive compulsive disorder, and insomnia.

Cyclothymia: A light version of bipolar including multiple mild episodes of hypomania and depressive symptoms that extend at least two years.

Deep brain stimulation (DBS): Electronic stimulation of targeted areas of the brain aimed at reducing bipolar depression symptoms.

Diagnostic and Statistical Manual of Mental Disorders (DSM): A textbook used by American psychiatrists that describes the criteria for diagnosing various mental illnesses.

Differential diagnosis: Distinguishing between two or more diseases or conditions that feature identical or similar symptoms.

Dopamine: A feel-good neurotransmitter that modulates attention, focus, and muscle movements.

Dysthymia: Chronic, low-level depression or persistent depressive disorder.

Electroconvulsive therapy (ECT): A medical procedure in which a low-level electrical current is applied to the brain to induce a mild seizure. ECT is used sparingly to treat deep depression.

Euthymic: Moods considered in the normal range—not manic.

Gamma-aminobutyric acid (GABA): An amino acid neurotransmitter that works mostly as an inhibitor or calming agent in the brain.

Glutamate: A neurotransmitter that's involved in revving up the central nervous system.

Hypersexual: Having an excessive interest or involvement in sexual activity.

Hyperthymic: High energy, highly extroverted, very physically and mentally active, highly confident, temperamental, stimulus seeking, and risk-taking.

Hypomania: Increased energy, having less need for sleep, and not manic.

Insight: Clear acceptance and understanding; the ability to objectively observe the behaviors and attitudes that are characteristic of bipolar disorder.

Life management team: Health-care professionals who work with the patient and the family to carry out treatment plans and make changes to those plans when symptoms indicate changes are needed.

Maintenance dose: Amount of medication intended to prevent the onset of symptoms rather than treat existing symptoms.

Major depressive episode: An extreme low mood that may last at least two weeks, characterized by despair, fatigue, loss or increase in appetite, loss of interest, and an increased need for sleep.

Mania: Extremely elevated mood characterized by euphoria, excessive energy, impulsivity, nervousness, impaired judgment, irritability, and a decreased need for sleep.

Mindfulness: A mental state of focusing on the present moment.

Mood chart: A graph showing the rise and fall of mood levels over time. Useful in predicting the onset of mood episodes and documenting responses to medications.

Mood stabilizer: Medication that reduces frequency or severity of episodes of depression or mania.

Neurons: Cells in the brain and nervous system that carry signals throughout the body.

Neurotransmitter: A chemical that's part of the communication systems between cells within the nervous system and from the nervous system to other parts of the body.

Omega-3: A source of several essential fatty acids. Some believe they are vital to the healthy development and function of the brain.

Phototherapy: The use of light to stimulate mood changes.

Presenting symptoms: Signs of discomfort that prompt a visit to a doctor.

Psychiatrist: A physician who specializes in the biology and physiology of the brain. A psychiatrist's role in treating bipolar includes diagnosis and medication prescription as well as patient education and psychotherapy.

Psychoeducation: A type of therapy that consists primarily of educating those affected about the condition, its causes, and its treatment, so they can more effectively manage the condition.

Psychologist: A doctor who plays a vital role in stabilizing moods by assessing brain functions and helping adjust negative thoughts, thought processes, and maladaptive behaviors.

Psychopharmacology: The study of the effects of medications on the brain.

Psychosis: Brain malfunction that blurs the line between real and imaginary, often causing delusions, auditory hallucinations, and irrational fears.

Psychotropic substance: Any chemical substance, usually a medicine, that affects mental functioning, emotions, or behavior.

Schizophrenia: A psychiatric disorder in which thought becomes dissociated from sensory input and emotions. Bipolar disorder is sometimes misdiagnosed as schizophrenia.

Self-medication: The attempt to stabilize moods by taking non-prescription chemical substances, including alcohol and marijuana, or by regulating doses of prescription medication without a doctor's assistance.

Stigmatize: To brand someone's behavior as disgraceful or shameful. There is a stigma attached to being bipolar.

Stressor: Anything that places demands on your brain and body. Stressors exacerbate bipolar highs and lows.

Support group: A group of patients or family members who meet in person or online to discuss and encourage one another in the face of a common illness like bipolar disorder.

Therapeutic level: The concentration of medicine required for medication to be effective.

Treatment plan: A complete explanation of the various materials, medications, and strategies used to treat bipolar disorder. These are outlined by the life management team. Treatment of bipolar disorder begins to bring a patient with mania or depression to symptomatic recovery. Once the patient is stable, the plan aims at reducing symptoms and preventing relapse.

About the Author

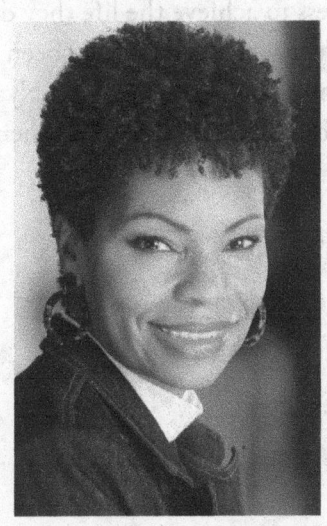

TAMU LEWIS, MBA, IS the cofounder and board president of the Lee Thompson Young Foundation. It is a nonprofit organization dedicated to helping erase the stigma associated with mental illness, advancing holistic health treatments, and improving the lives of all those impacted. She is also a mental health advocate, keynote speaker and HR leader.

Tamu launched the foundation as a living legacy to her brother, Lee, whom she lost to suicide in 2013. Knowing that her brother struggled with bipolar disorder and suffered in silence, Tamu is passionate about helping individuals cultivate emotional well-being for themselves and their loved ones. She is particularly dedicated to helping moms and their children.

Tamu has gained invaluable life lessons and practical solutions to help moms find a sense of relief, reclaim their joy, and optimize their mental wellness to achieve the life they desire and deserve.

For the past twenty-one years, she has been married to Stephen Lewis. She is the mom to two daughters, Nya (twenty) and Kai (eighteen). The family also includes Milo, their five-year-old dog.

www.ingramcontent.com/pod-product-compliance
Lightning Source LLC
Chambersburg PA
CBHW012224090425
24909CB00030B/257